7th CiiEM International Congress 2025—Empowering One Health to Reduce Social Vulnerabilities

7th CiiEM International Congress 2025—Empowering One Health to Reduce Social Vulnerabilities

Volume Editors

Ana I. Fernandes
João R. Vaz
Cristina Soeiro

MDPI

Basel • Beijing • Wuhan • Barcelona • Belgrade • Novi Sad • Cluj • Manchester

Volume Editors

Ana I. Fernandes
Egas Moniz School of Health & Science
Caparica
Portugal

João R. Vaz
Egas Moniz School of Health & Science
Caparica
Portugal

Cristina Soeiro
Egas Moniz School of Health & Science
Caparica
Portugal

Editorial Office
MDPI AG
Grosspeteranlage 5
4052 Basel, Switzerland

This is a reprint of the Proceedings, published open access by the journal *Medical Sciences Forum* (ISSN 2673-9992), freely accessible at: https://www.mdpi.com/2673-9992/37/1.

For citation purposes, cite each article independently as indicated on the article page online and as indicated below:

Lastname, A.A.; Lastname, B.B. Article Title. *Journal Name* **Year**, *Volume Number*, Page Range.

ISBN 978-3-7258-5631-2 (Hbk)
ISBN 978-3-7258-5632-9 (PDF)
https://doi.org/10.3390/books978-3-7258-5632-9

Cover image courtesy of João Tavares

Contents

About the Editors

Ana I. Fernandes

Ana I. Fernandes is an Associate Professor of Pharmaceutics and Head of the PharmSci Lab at the Egas Moniz School of Health & Science, Portugal. She graduated in Pharmaceutical Sciences (University of Lisbon, PT) and holds a PhD in Drug Delivery (University of London, UK). She has been involved in the study of polymers and polymeric systems with biomedical applications, namely, in the delivery of therapeutic proteins and conventional drugs. Her current research is related to formulations in pediatrics, drug solubility enhancement by co-amorphization, and the 3D printing of pharmaceuticals, as well as nutraceuticals and the usage of lifestyle drugs. Over the years, she has been the scientific advisor, principal investigator, or collaborator in several externally financed projects, a scientific consultant, and an Editorial Board Member and Guest Editor of several Special Issues of journals, and she has extensively published in international refereed journals. She served as President of the Scientific Committee of the 6th and 7th CiiEM Congresses.

João R. Vaz

João R. Vaz is an Associate Professor at the Egas Moniz School of Health & Science, where he also directs the Physiotherapy Department. He leads the Active Aging research group within the Egas Moniz Interdisciplinary Research Centre and coordinates the Integrative Movement for Networking Systems Laboratory. His research explores the intersection of human movement, rehabilitation, and dynamical systems and chaos theories. João has served as principal investigator and co-investigator on several nationally and internationally funded research projects and supervised more than 50 students from different educational levels in their research works: undergraduate (>25), master's (>15), and doctoral students (~10). His work integrates scientific research with clinical relevance, contributing to advancements in physiotherapy and movement sciences.

Cristina Soeiro

Cristina Soeiro holds a PhD in Justice Psychology from the University of Minho. She is an Associate Professor at the Egas Moniz University Institute (IUEM). Since 1990, she has been a Senior Specialist at the Institute of Judicial Police and Criminal Sciences, where she is responsible for the Psychology and Selection Office. She coordinates the Bachelor's Degree in Psychology and the Master's Degree in Forensic and Criminal Psychology at IUEM. She also leads the Integrative Research Group on Behaviour & Society at the Egas Moniz Center for Interdisciplinary Research (CiiEM). She serves as Vice-President of the Portuguese Association for Victim Support (APAV). She is a forensic expert witness in court in cases of homicide and sexual crimes. Her scientific research focuses on sexual offences and homicides within intimate relationships, as well as on arsonist behavior. She has published work on psychological profiling, homicide in intimate relationships, sexual abuse of children and adolescents, and typologies of forest arsonists, among other topics.

medical sciences forum

MDPI

Editorial

7th International Congress of CiiEM—Empowering One Health to Reduce Social Vulnerabilities

Ana I. Fernandes *, João R. Vaz and Cristina Soeiro

Egas Moniz Center for Interdisciplinary Research (CiiEM), Egas Moniz School of Health & Science, Monte de Caparica, 2829-511 Caparica, Portugal; jvaz@egasmoniz.edu.pt (J.R.V.); csoeiro@egasmoniz.edu.pt (C.S.)
* Correspondence: aifernandes@egasmoniz.edu.pt

1. Preface

Amidst the increasingly complex and interconnected challenges of our time, from climate change and emerging pandemics to deepening social inequalities, the One Health approach has gained renewed relevance as a guiding framework for research, policy, and practice [1,2]. By recognising that human, animal, and environmental health are inseparably linked, One Health promotes interdisciplinary collaboration and integrated strategies to build more resilient and inclusive societies [3,4].

The 7th CiiEM International Congress, under the theme "Empowering One Health to Reduce Social Vulnerabilities", held from 2 to 4 July 2025 in Caparica, Portugal, aimed to contribute meaningfully to this vision. Organised by the Egas Moniz Center for Interdisciplinary Research (CiiEM), the Congress gathered over 200 participants, bringing together researchers, practitioners, students, and stakeholders committed to transforming scientific knowledge into societal impact.

The invited speakers from leading institutions shared insights on the global and local challenges of applying One Health. These were strengthened by over 130 scientific contributions, presented as oral or poster communications, selected through a rigorous peer-review process. Particularly valuable were the contributions from students, whose enthusiasm and critical perspectives enriched the debates and demonstrated the vitality of the next generation of researchers.

Aligned with the Horizon Europe strategic plan (2025–2027) [5], the scientific programme reflected the urgency of applying a One Health lens today, covering topics such as technological innovation in biomedical research, digital inclusion, urban planning and public health, mental health and psychosocial resilience, sustainable food systems, antimicrobial resistance, and the social dimensions of healthcare access.

Beyond its scientific dimension, the congress also fulfilled an important pedagogical role. Many undergraduate and postgraduate students experienced, for the first time, what it means to be an author at a scientific event. They engaged directly with the processes of submission, revision, and editorial decisions, developing practical skills essential for their future academic and professional careers [6]. This hands-on experience not only demystified scientific publication but also fostered a critical understanding of quality, ethics, and scientific communication.

2. Statement of Peer Review

To ensure scientific quality and integrity, the congress followed a structured, two-phase editorial process. First, authors submitted abstracts (max. 500 words) which underwent blind peer review, ensuring impartiality and constructive feedback, coordinated by the

https://doi.org/10.3390/msf2025037016

Proceedings Editorial Board. In total, 143 abstracts were submitted, with 134 being accepted, reflecting an acceptance rate of 93.7%. Only accepted abstracts proceeded, optionally, to the submission of full proceedings papers (up to five pages), which were then subject to double peer review in the second phase. A total of 25 proceeding papers presented at the conference (5 oral and 20 poster communications) were accepted to be published in this dedicated volume of MDPI *Medical Sciences Forum*. Narrative literature reviews, study protocols, and systematic reviews without meta-analysis were not considered. A submission platform (Wordpress Plugin WP Abstracts Pro v.6.8.1 Abstracts & Manuscripts Submission, 2025) was used to manage the process.

Reviews were conducted by expert referees according to the professional and scientific standards expected of a proceedings journal. The evaluation considered several key criteria, as follows: (1) the aim, relevance, and originality of the work; (2) the quality and appropriateness of materials and methods; (3) ethical considerations; (4) scientific soundness and validity of results; and (5) the quality of writing, including clarity, text organisation, formatting, referencing, and English language and style. Reviewers provided constructive feedback, encouraging clarity and methodological rigour, particularly supporting students. Authors were notified of the reviewers' comments and invited to revise and resubmit their work through the platform. The Proceedings Editorial Board then reviewed the revised submissions, verified the corrections, and made the final decision. Authors were subsequently informed of the acceptance or rejection of their papers. The nominal list of those involved in the edition and reviewing process is included in the acknowledgements.

Finally, the volume editors also verified compliance with formatting guidelines and checked all submissions for plagiarism using Turnitin (www.turnitin.com; accessed on 21 July 2025) before finalising the papers for publication.

3. Thematic Clusters

The papers published in this volume illustrate the rich diversity and interdisciplinary focus of the 7th CiiEM International Congress. Organised around key themes that reflect the congress's mission to reduce social vulnerabilities through a One Health perspective, the volume begins with studies addressing public and global health, including medication safety, food supplement use, and breastfeeding practices.

A second cluster of papers delves into forensic science and psychology, exploring topics such as intimate partner violence, sexual harassment, and innovative forensic techniques applied to neurological conditions like Parkinson's disease.

Education and pedagogical research feature strongly, with studies analysing curriculum innovation, science teaching models, and student attitudes toward community service and reintegration initiatives.

The volume also highlights rehabilitation and physiotherapy, presenting clinical case studies and strategies like robotic gait training, kinesiotaping, and online rehabilitation for chronic conditions, alongside studies on compassion fatigue and the physiology of elite sports.

In oral health and dentistry, papers examine patient attitudes to laser technology, the treatment of xerostomia, and material degradation in orthodontics, as well as diagnostic delays in burning mouth syndrome.

Cutting-edge artificial intelligence methods applied to cancer prognosis and studies in hospital emergency care further illustrate the congress's breadth, combining clinical research, digital tools, and patient-centred perspectives.

4. Closing Remarks

The One Health approach offers a powerful framework for emphasising collaboration across disciplines and sectors. The contributions published here reflect the congress's interdisciplinary and pedagogical spirit, offering innovative research grounded in real-world applications and a shared commitment to improving health outcomes across human, animal, and environmental domains. We hope this publication serves not only as a scientific record but also as an inspiration for future research and action towards a healthier, fairer, and more sustainable world.

Acknowledgments: We are grateful to the Proceedings Editorial Board and the reviewers listed in the Appendix A who generously shared their expertise, contributing significantly to the scientific quality and rigour of the studies published here. Special thanks to the team responsible for the management and maintenance of the congress website and submission platform, secretarial work, and creative input.

Conflicts of Interest: The authors declare no conflict of interest.

Appendix A

References

1. Lerner, H.; Berg, C. The concept of health in One Health and some practical implications for research and education: What is One Health? *Infect. Ecol. Epidemiol.* **2015**, *5*, 25300. [CrossRef]
2. Destoumieux-Garzón, D.; Mavingui, P.; Boetsch, G.; Boissier, J.; Darriet, F.; Duboz, P.; Fritsch, C.; Giraudoux, P.; Le Roux, F.; Morand, S.; et al. The One Health concept: 10 years old and a long road ahead. *Front. Vet. Sci.* **2018**, *5*, 14. [CrossRef]
3. Pitt, S.J.; Gunn, A. The One Health concept. *Br. J. Biomed. Sci.* **2024**, *81*, 12366. [CrossRef] [PubMed]
4. One Health. Available online: https://www.who.int/news-room/fact-sheets/detail/one-health (accessed on 14 July 2025).

5. European Commission: Directorate-General for Research and Innovation. *Horizon Europe strategic Plan 2025–2027*; Publications Office of the European Union: Luxembourg, 2024. [CrossRef]
6. OECD. *The Future of Education and Skills: Education 2030*; Organisation for Economic Co-Operation and Development: Paris, France, 2018.

medical sciences forum

MDPI

Proceeding Paper

A One Health Perspective on the Clinical, Behavioural, and Environmental Risks of Chronic Proton Pump Inhibitor Use in Older Adults †

Maria Deolinda Auxtero

Egas Moniz Center for Interdisciplinary Research (CiiEM); Egas Moniz School of Health & Science, Caparica, 2829-511 Almada, Portugal; mauxtero@egasmoniz.edu.pt

† Presented at the 7th CiiEM International Congress 2025—Empowering One Health to Reduce Social Vulnerabilities, Caparica, Portugal, 2–4 July 2025.

Abstract: This study explores the clinical, behavioural, and environmental risks of chronic proton pump inhibitor (PPI) use in older adults through a One Health perspective. Among 246 participants, 32.5% were receiving PPI therapy, with 91.3% on long-term treatment, frequently lacking clear clinical justification. Polypharmacy, drug interactions, and risky lifestyle behaviours were common. Environmental review highlighted the potential persistence of PPI transformation products in water systems, raising concerns about ecological impact and antimicrobial resistance. These findings underscore the urgency of implementing deprescribing strategies, enhancing patient education, and adopting sustainable prescribing practices that align human and environmental health.

Keywords: One Health; proton pump inhibitors; elderly; polypharmacy; environmental contaminants

1. Introduction

The One Health philosophy—emphasising the interconnectedness of human, animal, and environmental health—provides a robust framework for addressing complex, multifactorial health issues. This is especially relevant to vulnerable populations, such as older adults, who face heightened risks due to ageing, multimorbidity, and polypharmacy. Proton pump inhibitors (PPIs), commonly used in this group for acid-related gastrointestinal illness, are effective in the short-term but increasingly controversial when used long-term due to their adverse effects and questionable prescribing practices [1]. Aligned with One Health principles, this study considers not only individual-level clinical and behavioural risks but also the broader environmental implications at the system level of chronic PPI use.

Global data show that 25% of PPI users remain on treatment for over a year, and nearly a third for more than three years—often without clinical justification [2]. In older adults, prolonged PPI use has been linked to nutrient malabsorption, fractures, kidney disease, and cognitive decline [2,3]. These risks are compounded by behavioural and therapeutic inertia [3], the lack of deprescribing guidelines, and the limited uptake of structured interventions. The C-SENIoR trial, a pragmatic study conducted in Portugal, showed the feasibility and value of collaborative, pharmacist-led deprescribing in primary care [4].

From a One Health standpoint, the implications go beyond individual health. Inappropriate prescribing, including PPI, contributes to healthcare overuse, pharmaceutical waste, and environmental contamination via excreted drug residues entering water systems [5]. These can disrupt aquatic ecosystems, underscoring the need for sustainable prescribing practices.

This work adopts a One Health perspective in addressing the clinical, behavioural, and environmental risks of chronic PPI use in older adults. Drawing on cohort data and the current literature, we aim to identify systemic vulnerabilities and propose cross-disciplinary strategies—such as deprescribing, patient education, and policy-level action—to support safer, more sustainable care.

2. Materials and Methods

This repeated cross-sectional study involved two independent cohorts of community-dwelling adults aged 65 and older, assessed in 2023/2024 and 2024/2025 under the ESPIEM (Healthy Ageing—Egas Moniz Interdisciplinary Project). Although the same protocol was used, each cohort comprised a distinct sample. A convenience sample of individuals taking at least two medications was recruited by third-year pharmacy students via personal networks. Participants were eligible for inclusion if they were aged 65 years or older, lived in the community, were taking two or more medications, and were able to provide informed consent. Individuals were excluded if they had cognitive impairment that interfered with consent, were living in institutional care settings, or declined to participate. Data were collected through structured interviews, medication reviews, and lifestyle surveys. Pharmacological risk was assessed using the Medscape Drug Interaction Checker [6]. Lifestyle factors included smoking, alcohol and caffeine consumption, and sunscreen use. Descriptive statistics (frequencies, percentages, means) summarised PPI use and drug interaction risk. Data from both years (n = 246 elderly individuals; 144 in 2023/2024, 102 in 2024/2025) were pooled to describe pharmacotherapy patterns and health behaviours.

As no primary environmental sampling was performed, a focused narrative literature review was conducted to explore the potential environmental risks of chronic pharmaceutical contaminants, with particular emphasis on PPIs and their transformation products in wastewater and surface waters. These findings were qualitatively integrated to inform the ecological implications within a One Health perspective.

3. Results and Discussion

3.1. Participant Profile and PPI Use

Among the 246 participants (mean age: 76.6 years), 80 individuals (32.5%) were receiving PPI therapy. The most commonly prescribed PPI was esomeprazole, followed by pantoprazole and omeprazole (Table 1). Of the PPI users, 73 (91.3%) had been on treatment for more than six months.

Table 1. Summary of PPI use, drug interactions, and lifestyle factors among older adults (n = 80).

Category	Number (n)	Percentage (%)
Total PPI users	80	100
Sex distribution (PPI users)		
Women	45	56.2
Men	35	43.8
Long-term PPI use (>6 months)	73	91.3

Table 1. *Cont.*

Category	Number (*n*)	Percentage (%)
PPI name (dosage)		
Esomeprazole (20–40 mg)	26	32.5
Pantoprazole (20–40 mg)	24	30.0
Omeprazole (20 mg)	22	27.5
Lansoprazole (15–30 mg)	7	8.8
Rabeprazole (10 mg)	1	1.3
Drug interactions		
Serious [1]	25	31.3
Monitor Closely [1]	56	70
Lifestyle behaviours		
Daily alcohol consumption	43	53.8
Active smoking	5	6.3
Regular coffee intake	47	58.8
Infrequent or no sunscreen use	72	90.0
Healthcare context		
Has family doctor	67	83.8
Concomitant medications (mean)	7.5	-
Source of the PPI prescription		
Family doctor	47	58.8
Other doctor	32	40.0
Pharmacist	1	1.2

[1] Number of PPI users with 'Serious' or 'Monitor Closely' drug interactions.

Polypharmacy was common among PPI users, who were taking an average of 7.5 medications concurrently. A pharmacological review identified 293 'Monitor Closely' drug interactions, affecting 70% of PPI users, and 48 'Serious' interactions (31.3%). One of the 'Serious' interactions involved a PPI (omeprazole) and clopidogrel. Additionally, 28.8% of patients on PPIs were also prescribed corticosteroids, non-steroidal anti-inflammatories, or other drugs associated with gastric toxicity, potentially justifying PPI co-prescription but also underscoring the need for regular benefit–risk assessments. In elderly patients, age-related pharmacokinetic changes increase the likelihood of adverse outcomes from prolonged PPI use, including nutrient malabsorption, increased infection risk, and potentially even cognitive decline [1]. Importantly, PPIs are photosensitising drugs that may contribute to UV-induced skin damage [7]. Yet, in our analysis, 90% of users reported rarely or never using sunscreen, revealing a gap in preventive education. Lifestyle analysis revealed further behavioural risk factors: 6.25% of users were current smokers, 58.8% consumed coffee regularly, and 53.8% consumed alcohol—all of which can worsen gastrointestinal symptoms or alter drug metabolism, potentially prolonging or complicating treatment. Despite 83.8% of PPI users having a designated family doctor, the data suggest limited therapeutic reassessment and little emphasis on behavioural counselling, representing missed opportunities for deprescribing and lifestyle optimisation.

These findings reflect a broader trend of long-term PPI overuse globally, often extending beyond the recommended 4–8 week course typically advised for conditions like gastroesophageal reflux disease. In our cohort, 91.3% of PPI users had been on therapy for more than six months, underscoring persistent therapeutic inertia. This aligns with recent findings from a 2025 evaluation of primary care practices in England, where 62% of patients on continuous PPI therapy had no recorded indication, and 99% of those with short-term indications exceeded the recommended duration of use [8].

This highlights the need for greater awareness, regular treatment reassessment, and the implementation of structured deprescribing strategies. A 2024 scoping review emphasised that most interventions targeting inappropriate PPI use rely on education and enablement strategies, with pharmacist-led reviews and algorithm-based tools showing the most consistent effectiveness [9]. Notably, 58.8% of PPIs in our study were prescribed by family doctors, positioning primary care settings as key leverage points for intervention and change. The absence of regular medication reviews, even among patients with routine access to healthcare, reveals systemic shortcomings in care continuity. Addressing both reflective and impulsive behavioural determinants—such as beliefs about medication necessity and habitual prescribing—has been recommended to improve deprescribing outcomes [9]. Integrating pharmacists into geriatric assessments, fostering shared decision-making, and equipping clinicians to discuss lifestyle-related risk factors—such as alcohol use, photoprotection, and dietary triggers—are essential steps to improve outcomes. Given the known photosensitising potential of PPIs, photoprotection counselling should become a routine part of care [7].

3.2. Ecological Considerations

Although our primary data did not include environmental sampling, we conducted a focused review of the environmental science literature to contextualise the ecological implications of chronic PPI use within a One Health framework. From this perspective, the clinical and behavioural challenges discussed above are intrinsically linked to environmental concerns. While PPIs are widely prescribed, their direct detection in surface waters has been limited due to extensive human metabolism and rapid abiotic degradation. However, recent studies have shown that omeprazole, one of the most commonly used PPIs, can undergo photodegradation and hydrolysis in aquatic environments, forming several transformation products (TPs) that may persist for longer than the parent compound [10,11]. Photodegradation experiments in various water types (distilled, river, lake, and seawater) showed that natural constituents such as dissolved organic matter and nitrate ions influence the degradation rate of omeprazole. Seven TPs were identified, some also formed via hydrolysis. These were detected in both influent and effluent samples from wastewater treatment plants, suggesting that conventional treatment processes may not fully remove them. Notably, some TPs appeared more frequently than the parent compound, indicating that environmental monitoring efforts should prioritise these derivatives [11]. Toxicity testing using *Vibrio fischeri* revealed that while omeprazole itself exhibits high acute toxicity, its photodegradation products are significantly less toxic, suggesting solar photolysis may reduce environmental risk. Nevertheless, the presence of multiple TPs and their potential bioactivity highlight the need for further ecotoxicological evaluation. The persistence of PPIs and their TPs in surface waters may contribute not only to aquatic toxicity but also to the spread of antimicrobial resistance, particularly when residues interact with other pharmaceutical pollutants [5].

This study's limitations include convenience sampling, recall bias from self-reported data, and the lack of primary environmental sampling, which limits generalisability and prevents direct ecological assessment. Nonetheless, the literature review offers a meaningful basis for future environmental research.

4. Conclusions

This study highlights the complex risks of chronic PPI use in older adults. Clinically, the high prevalence of long-term use, polypharmacy, and serious drug interactions calls for regular medication reviews and appropriate deprescribing. Behavioural factors—such as poor sunscreen use, alcohol and caffeine intake, and continued smoking—reflect missed opportunities for patient education. These issues are compounded by the environmental impact of PPI residues and TPs in wastewater, reinforcing the need for prescribing practices that support both human and ecological health. Recommendations include incorporating environmental considerations into clinical guidelines, promoting photoprotection, and empowering primary care to reduce unnecessary drug exposure. Advancing eco-pharmacovigilance and cross-sector collaboration is key to sustainable prescribing.

A One Health–oriented approach must integrate medication review, lifestyle counselling, and environmental awareness to reduce risk and promote more sustainable, person-centred care. Future research should directly investigate the environmental presence and ecotoxicity of TPs derived from PPIs through primary sampling and experimental models.

Funding: This research was funded by Egas Moniz, Cooperativa de Ensino Superior—Envelhecimento Saudável—Projeto Interdisciplinar Egas Moniz (ESPIEM), 2022. The author also thanks FCT/MCTES for the financial support to CiiEM (10.54499/UIDB/04585/2020) through national funds.

Institutional Review Board Statement: This study was conducted in accordance with the Declaration of Helsinki, and approved by the Ethics Committee of Egas Moniz (file no. 12/30, 25 May 2023).

Informed Consent Statement: Informed consent was obtained from all subjects involved in the study.

Data Availability Statement: The raw data supporting the conclusions of this article will be made available by the authors on request.

Acknowledgments: The author thanks 2023–2024 and 2024–2025 third-year pharmacy students at Egas Moniz for their assistance with data collection.

Conflicts of Interest: The author declares no conflicts of interest.

References

1. Freedberg, D.E.; Kim, L.S.; Yang, Y.-X. The risks and benefits of long-term use of proton pump inhibitors: Expert review and best practice advice from the American Gastroenterological Association. *Gastroenterology* **2017**, *152*, 706–715. [CrossRef] [PubMed]
2. Shanika, L.G.T.; Reynolds, A.; Pattison, S.; Braund, R. Proton pump inhibitor use: Systematic review of global trends and practices. *Eur. J. Clin. Pharmacol.* **2023**, *79*, 1159–1172. [CrossRef] [PubMed]
3. Dutta, A.K.; Jain, A.; Jearth, V.; Mahajan, R.; Panigrahi, M.K.; Sharma, V.; Goenka, M.K.; Kochhar, R.; Makharia, G.; Reddy, D.N.; et al. Guidelines on optimizing the use of proton pump inhibitors: PPI stewardship. *Indian J. Gastroenterol.* **2023**, *42*, 601–628. [CrossRef] [PubMed]
4. Romano, S.; Monteiro, L.; Guerreiro, J.P.; Simões, J.B.; Rodrigues, A.T.; Lunet, N.; Perelman, J. Effectiveness and cost-effectiveness of a collaborative deprescribing intervention of proton-pump-inhibitors on community-dwelling older adults: Protocol for the C-SENIoR, a pragmatic non-randomized controlled trial. *PLoS ONE* **2024**, *19*, e0298181. [CrossRef] [PubMed]
5. Jani, M.; Kumari, S. Pharmaceutical Wastewater and Environmental Contamination: Challenges, Innovations, and Future Directions. *PEXACY Int. J. Pharm. Sci.* **2024**, *3*, 79–98. [CrossRef]
6. Drug Interactions Checker—Medscape Drug Reference Database. Available online: https://reference.medscape.com/drug-interactionchecker (accessed on 9 August 2023).
7. Alrashidi, A.; Rhodes, L.E.; Sharif, J.C.H.; Kreeshan, F.C.; Farrar, M.D.; Ahad, T. Systemic drug photosensitivity-Culprits, impact and investigation in 122 patients. *Photodermatol. Photoimmunol. Photomed.* **2020**, *36*, 441–451. [CrossRef] [PubMed]
8. Plehhova, K.; Wray, J.; Aluko, P.; Sutton, S.; McArdle, J.; Dawson, A.; Coyle, C.; Stevens, R.M. Prescribing practices for proton pump inhibitors among primary care physicians in England: An evaluation. *BJGP Open* **2025**, *9*, BJGPO.2024.0059. [CrossRef] [PubMed]
9. van Gestel, L.C.; Adriaanse, M.A.; Kanis, S.L.; Mensink-Bout, S.M.; Schoones, J.W.; Numans, M.E.; Kiefte-de Jong, J.C.; van den Brink, G. Determinants of and interventions for Proton Pump Inhibitor prescription behavior: A systematic scoping review. *BMC Prim. Care* **2024**, *25*, 208. [CrossRef] [PubMed]

10. Kosma, C.I.; Lambropoulou, D.A.; Albanis, T.A. Analysis, occurrence, fate and risks of proton pump inhibitors, their metabolites and transformation products in aquatic environment: A review. *Sci. Total Environ.* **2016**, *569–570*, 732–750. [CrossRef] [PubMed]
11. Kosma, C.I.; Lambropoulou, D.A.; Albanis, T.A. Photochemical transformation and wastewater fate and occurrence of omeprazole: HRMS for elucidation of transformation products and target and suspect screening analysis in wastewaters. *Sci. Total Environ.* **2017**, *590–591*, 592–601. [CrossRef] [PubMed]

medical sciences forum

MDPI

Proceeding Paper

Pharmaceutical Profiling of Fentanyl Use in Portugal: Consumption Patterns and Abuse Deterrence Gaps †

Ana Isabel Fernandes

Egas Moniz Center for Interdisciplinary Research (CiiEM), Egas Moniz School of Health & Science, Monte de Caparica, 2829-511 Caparica, Portugal; aifernandes@egasmoniz.edu.pt

† Presented at the 7th CiiEM International Congress 2025—Empowering One Health to Reduce Social Vulnerabilities, Caparica, Portugal, 2–4 July 2025.

Abstract: Fentanyl, a potent synthetic opioid used in pain management, has seen a marked rise in outpatient use in Portugal between 2015 and 2022. During this period, consumption nearly doubled, with transdermal patches and sublingual tablets dominating the market. Rapid-onset formulations lacking abuse-deterrent features pose have heightened the risks of misuse and diversion. Despite these concerns, no abuse-deterrent fentanyl products are currently available in Portugal. These findings expose critical regulatory and pharmaceutical gaps. To mitigate public health and environmental risks, a coordinated strategy—encompassing prescription monitoring, education, safer formulations, and a One Health approach—is urgently needed to ensure responsible opioid use and stewardship.

Keywords: fentanyl; dosage forms; abuse-deterrent formulations; drug abuse potential; Portugal

1. Introduction

Fentanyl, a synthetic opioid approximately 50–100 times more potent than morphine, has become a cornerstone in the management of severe pain, particularly in oncological settings and perioperative care [1]. Despite its therapeutic utility, fentanyl's pharmacokinetic profile—characterized by high lipid solubility, rapid central nervous system penetration, and potent μ-opioid receptor agonism—renders it especially susceptible to misuse, dependence, and fatal overdose [2].

Globally, the surge in fentanyl-related morbidity and mortality has prompted urgent policy and surveillance responses, particularly in North America, where the non-medical use of illicitly manufactured fentanyl has driven a public health crisis [3,4]. In contrast, until recently, in countries like Portugal, fentanyl was predominantly accessed through legal prescriptions for legitimate medical purposes. Nonetheless, signs of rising consumption and concern over abuse potential have emerged [5]. Illicit production and use, the diversion and misuse of medicines, and the online sale of non-controlled new psychoactive substances is a reality in Europe [6].

The pharmacological and physicochemical properties of fentanyl dosage forms strongly influence their potential for misuse. Immediate-release products offer rapid onset and are often associated with higher abuse liability, while extended-release systems, although intended for steady delivery, may still be tampered with in order to extract the drug [7]. To address these concerns, the development of abuse-deterrent formulations (ADFs) has gained traction—particularly in the United States—as a harm-reduction strategy. Despite progress in this area, ADFs remain underutilized or unavailable in many European markets [8]. These technologies incorporate various deterrent mechanisms, including prodrugs, aversive agents, opioid antagonists, or physical and chemical barriers that inhibit common manipulation methods such as crushing, dissolving, or snorting [7].

This study aims to characterize the pharmaceutical landscape of fentanyl in Portugal, with particular attention being paid to dosage form distribution, consumption trends, and formulation-related abuse potential. By identifying current gaps in abuse deterrence, this research seeks to inform future strategies for safer opioid prescribing, surveillance, and pharmaceutical innovation in the Portuguese context.

2. Materials and Methods

Sales data (expressed as number of packages) for all analgesic opioids dispensed in community pharmacies in Portugal between 2015 and 2022 were obtained from the National Pharmacies Association (Associação Nacional das Farmácias—ANF). The total number of doses was calculated by multiplying the number of packages by the corresponding unit quantity per package. Data were cross-checked and validated with information available from the Infarmed database [9] to sort for potential inconsistencies. Data regarding fentanyl for injection or perfusion used in hospital settings under medical supervision were not considered. The following variables were extracted and classified for analysis: year of dispensing, dosage form, potency, and brand vs. generic status. To assess the potential for misuse or abuse, each dosage form was categorized based on evidence from the literature and the pharmaceutical and pharmacokinetic profile of the product, considering characteristics such as route of administration, onset of action, and tamperability. Descriptive statistics were used to quantify and report annual consumption by opioid type and dosage form, identify consumption trends over time, and contextualize these trends with respect to abuse potential.

3. Results and Discussion

This retrospective observational study aimed to characterize fentanyl consumption in Portugal over an eight-year period (2015–2022). The analysis included all legally dispensed analgesic opioid medicines used in ambulatory settings (Figure 1).

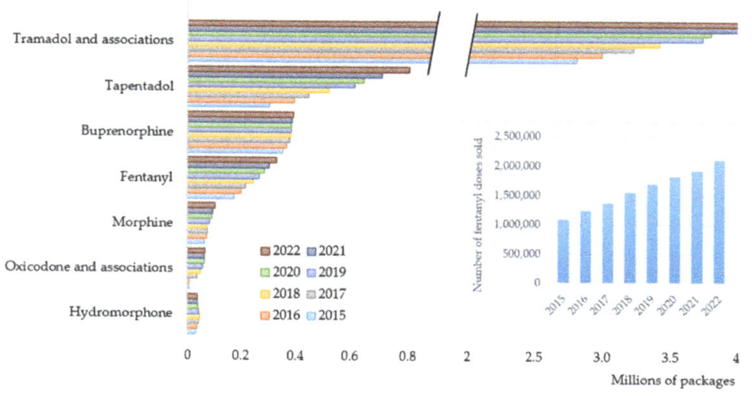

Figure 1. Number of packages of opioid analgesics sold in community pharmacies in Portugal (2015–2022), highlighting the steady increase in consumption. Note that the scale has been broken for clarity. The insert shows the sales of fentanyl in number of doses over the same time.

Fentanyl ranked as the fourth most consumed opioid in Portugal, following tramadol (and its fixed-dose combinations), tapentadol, and buprenorphine. Over the study period, fentanyl consumption nearly doubled, increasing by approximately 90% both in terms of packages and doses sold (Figure 1 and insert). A linear upward trend was observed, with an average annual increase of approximately 22,468 packages/year. The consistent annual growth in fentanyl use emphasizes its increasing role in pain management, despite the availability of alternative analgesics. Remarkably, the rate of increase in fentanyl use outpaced that of traditional strong opioids such as morphine and hydromorphone, suggesting a preferential shift toward fentanyl formulations, possibly due to its high potency, availability of various non-invasive administration routes, and extended-release dosage forms.

A gradual increase in the generic-to-brand ratio was observed both in terms of the number of packages sold and total doses consumed, indicating a growing penetration of generic fentanyl products in the Portuguese ambulatory market. This trend aligns with national and European policies promoting generic use as a cost-containment measure.

Figure 2 illustrates the share of fentanyl dosage forms sold (in number of doses), emphasizing the predominance of transdermal patches and sublingual tablets, which together consistently account for most of the total fentanyl use throughout the study period. Constant transdermal consumption (58–60%) reflects its established role in chronic pain management, particularly in oncology and palliative care. Sublingual tablets show a notable upward trend, increasing from 27.45% in 2015 to 36.58% in 2022. On the other hand, oral transmucosal lozenges showed a significant decrease from 11.66% in 2015 to 2.81% in 2022. This downward trend might reflect reduced prescribing due to concerns over misuse or risk to children, as they look like lollipops. Buccal films and nasal sprays (introduced in 2019) represent marginal shares of overall consumption, respectively, 0.56 and 0.20% in 2022. This is attributable to factors such as limited prescriber familiarity, higher costs, recent market entry, specialized therapeutic indications, and restricted access. Notably, the three least consumed are exclusively available as brand-name medicines.

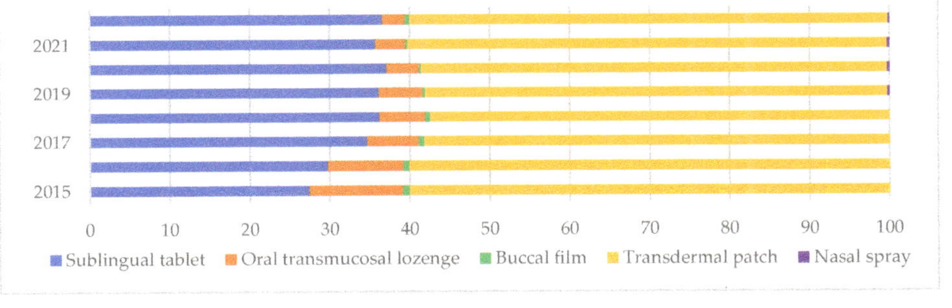

Figure 2. Percentage of fentanyl doses sold in community pharmacies in Portugal between 2015 and 2022, categorized by dosage form.

Dosage forms that are rapid-acting, highly potent, and approved for outpatient use present an increased risk of non-medical use, diversion, and accidental exposure, particularly within household settings. Therefore, identifying the key factors potentially contributing to the risk of misuse and abuse is essential. Table 1 presents a comparative overview of fentanyl dosage forms authorized in Portugal, summarizing their pharmacokinetic profiles, route of administration, and associated abuse deterrence and potential.

Table 1. Pharmaceutical typification of fentanyl dosage forms currently available in Portugal regarding abuse potential [2,8–10].

Dosage Form	Route	Potency	Onset	Duration	ADF	Abuse Potential
Patch	Transdermal	12.5–100 μg/h [1]	Slow	Long	No[2]	Low to Moderate [2]
Sublingual tablet	Sublingual	100–800 μg	Fast	Short	No	High
Buccal film	Oromucosal	200–800 μg	Fast	Short	No	High
Lozenge with applicator	Oromucosal	200–800 μg	Fast	Short	No	High
Nasal spray	Intranasal	100–400 μg/dose	Fast	Short	No	High
Injectable solutions	Intravenous	0.05 mg/mL	Immediate	Short	No	Moderate [3] to High [4]

ADF—Abuse Deterrent Formulation. [1] Corresponding to a total of 2.1–16.8 mg of fentanyl per patch. [2] Partial deterrence, considering matrix patches (e.g., Durogesic®), from which it is difficult to extract the drug; potential for misuse via extraction or reuse. [3] Parenteral forms under restricted access. [4] Injectable forms have immediate bioavailability, increasing the risk of overdose if diverted for non-medical use.

Currently, fentanyl ADFs are unavailable in Portugal. Among the existing options, transdermal patches—despite containing high total amounts of fentanyl (up to 16.8 mg per unit)—exhibit a slow onset and prolonged duration of action, which, in combination with partial tamper-resistance in matrix-based systems, contributes to a comparatively lower risk of misuse under normal therapeutic conditions. While not formally classified as ADFs, matrix patches offer some deterrence, since drug extraction is significantly more difficult than using reservoir-type systems. However, methods of tampering (drug extraction and intravenous or inhalation use) and misuse after disposal (oral, transmucosal, rectal use of whole patch) have been reported [11]. These risks underline the need for improved safeguards in fentanyl delivery systems to reduce diversion and non-medical use.

In contrast, rapid-onset formulations—such as sublingual tablets, buccal films, oromucosal lozenges, and nasal sprays—have fast systemic absorption and short durations, which are characteristics that increase their appeal for non-medical use. These formulations lack abuse-deterrent features and are often prescribed in outpatient settings, intensifying the risk. Injectable forms, although restricted to hospital use, have immediate bioavailability and high potency. While their accessibility is limited, they present a significant risk if diverted due to the high potential for overdose.

Overall, the formulation characteristics—particularly route of administration, onset of action, and presence or absence of abuse-deterrent features—play a critical role in determining the misuse liability of fentanyl products. These insights reinforce the importance of monitoring not only total consumption, but also the distribution by dosage form, identifying those incorporating strategies to mitigate opioid-related harms.

Although limited due to the lack of data on hospital use and the inability to directly distinguish misuse from legitimate prescribing, the growing outpatient use of fentanyl is noted. This aspect, in the absence of ADFs, reveals a critical gap in Portugal's pharmaceutical and regulatory strategies, which may facilitate non-medical use or unintentional misuse. To address this, several targeted measures should be considered. First, the inclusion of fentanyl ADFs in national formularies to promote safer prescribing. Improved surveillance systems that integrate prescription data with real-world usage are also essential for detecting emerging misuse patterns. Education programs for healthcare professionals and patients should emphasize safe storage, proper disposal, and early identification of misuse. Also, regulatory bodies should encourage or mandate pharmaceutical manufacturers to adopt abuse-deterrent packaging and delivery technologies.

Fentanyl use also poses broader risks across the One Health spectrum. Improper disposal of fentanyl products may result in accidental exposure to animals and environmental contamination, while veterinary use—although limited—still presents diversion risks. Coordinated action across sectors is vital: prescription monitoring, environmental surveillance, and secure veterinary practices must work in concert. Cross-sectoral collaboration is essential to mitigate these interconnected risks and ensure the sustainable and responsible use of fentanyl.

4. Conclusions

The predominance of transdermal and sublingual forms, both of which carry moderate-to-high abuse potential, highlights the need for continued pharmacovigilance and prescriber education. The overall rise in fentanyl use highlights its increasing role in pain therapy, but also amplifies the urgency for implementing ADFs, particularly in formulations with rapid onset. A comprehensive opioid stewardship model with One Health alignment should be implemented.

Funding: A.I.F. thanks FCT/MCTES for the financial support to CiiEM (10.54499/UIDB/04585/2020) through national funds.

Institutional Review Board Statement: This study used publicly available and anonymized aggregated data and did not require ethical approval. No patient-identifiable data were accessed.

Informed Consent Statement: Not applicable.

Data Availability Statement: The raw data supporting the conclusions of this article will be made available by the authors on request.

Acknowledgments: The author gratefully acknowledges Zilda Mendes from the Centre for Health Evaluation & Research (ANF) for kindly providing access to the consumption data.

Conflicts of Interest: The author declares no conflicts of interest.

References

1. Volkow, N.D.; Jones, E.B.; Einstein, E.B.; Wargo, E.M. Prevention and treatment of opioid misuse and addiction: A review. *JAMA Psychiatry* **2019**, *76*, 208–216. [CrossRef] [PubMed]
2. Gudin, J.A.; Nalamachu, S.; Leong, M.; Schatman, M. Abuse potential of fentanyl and its analogs. *J. Pain Res.* **2020**, *13*, 1223–1230.
3. World Drug Report 2023. Available online: https://www.unodc.org/unodc/en/data-and-analysis/world-drug-report-2023.html (accessed on 21 May 2025).
4. CDC Synthetic Opioids Overdose Data. Available online: https://www.cdc.gov/nchs/nvss/vsrr/drug-overdose-data.htm (accessed on 22 May 2025).
5. Carmona Araújo, A.; Guerreiro, J.P.; Bulhosa, C.; Alves da Costa, F.; Goulão, J.; Martins, A.P. Use and misuse of psychoactive medicines: A descriptive cross-sectional study in a densely populated region of Portugal. *J. Pharm. Policy Pract.* **2024**, *17*, 2369319. [CrossRef] [PubMed]
6. Mounteney, J.; Giraudon, I.; Denissov, G.; Griffiths, P. Fentanyls: Are we missing the signs? Highly potent and on the rise in Europe. *Int. J. Drug Policy* **2015**, *26*, 626–631. [CrossRef] [PubMed]
7. Chandegra, B.; Raval, J.; Prajapati, P. A review on advanced formulations strategies to prevent prescription drug abuse and their impact. *Discov. Med.* **2024**, *1*, 123. [CrossRef]
8. FDA. *Abuse-Deterrent Opioids—Evaluation and Labeling Guidance for Industry*; U.S. Food and Drug Administration: Silver Spring, MD, USA, 2022.
9. Infomed. Available online: https://extranet.infarmed.pt/INFOMED-fo/ (accessed on 22 May 2025).
10. Cicero, T.J.; Ellis, M.S.; Kasper, Z.A. Relative preferences in abuse of immediate-release versus extended-release opioids in a sample of treatment-seeking individuals. *Drug Alcohol Depend.* **2017**, *177*, 105–110.
11. Kuczyńska, K.; Grzonkowski, P.; Kacprzak, Ł.; Zawilska, J.B. Abuse of fentanyl: An emerging problem to face. *Forensic Sci. Int.* **2018**, *289*, 207–214. [CrossRef] [PubMed]

medical sciences forum

MDPI

Proceeding Paper

Patterns of Supplement Consumption and Interaction Risks Among Polymedicated Older Adults: A Descriptive Study †

Maria Deolinda Auxtero * and Ana Isabel Fernandes *

Egas Moniz Center for Interdisciplinary Research (CiiEM), Egas Moniz School of Health & Science, Monte de Caparica, 2829-511 Caparica, Portugal
* Correspondence: mauxtero@egasmoniz.edu.pt (M.D.A.); aifernandes@egasmoniz.edu.pt (A.I.F.)
† Presented at the 7th CiiEM International Congress 2025—Empowering One Health to Reduce Social Vulnerabilities, Caparica, Portugal, 2–4 July 2025.

Abstract: This study investigates the use of food supplements (FS) among polymedicated elderly individuals and assesses potential FS–drug interaction risks. A total of 98 community-dwelling older adults were surveyed and 18.4% reported FS use. FS were mostly used for musculoskeletal and cognitive support, with 71% having potential metabolic interactions via CYP enzymes or P-glycoprotein. Monthly costs reached €55. The findings reveal a complex interaction landscape and financial burden, underscoring the need for medication reviews and health literacy efforts to ensure safer FS use in older adults. This study aligns with One Health principles by linking clinical, social, and economic aspects of aging.

Keywords: polypharmacy; food supplements; drug–supplement interactions; geriatric pharmacotherapy; One Health

1. Introduction

The aging population is experiencing a marked increase in chronic conditions, often requiring the use of multiple medications—a phenomenon known as polypharmacy. Among older adults, defined commonly as individuals aged 65 years and above, polypharmacy is a growing concern due to its association with adverse drug events, hospitalizations, and reduced quality of life [1,2]. In parallel, there is a rising trend in the use of food supplements (FS), such as vitamins, minerals, and herbal products, often taken without professional guidance [3]. The use of FS by elderly polymedicated individuals raises concerns that go beyond pharmacological safety. Because these products are not classified as medicines, they fall outside reimbursement systems and regulatory frameworks, placing the full financial burden on users. For older adults, many of whom live on limited incomes, this can deepen existing social vulnerabilities and contribute to health inequities.

Due to the natural origin, FS are often perceived as inherently safe, but their concomitant use with prescription medications can lead to clinically significant interactions [4,5]. Older adults are particularly vulnerable due to age-related changes in drug disposition, along with the cumulative effects of polypharmacy [6]. Notably, FS such as St. John's Wort, *Ginkgo biloba*, or calcium can interfere with drug absorption or metabolism, risking therapeutic failure or toxicity [7]. Others, such as Ephedra (banned in Europe and US but available through the internet), Yohymbe (*Pausinystalia yohimbe*), Kava (*Piper methysticum*), or green tea extract, can lead to potentially fatal outcomes, especially when used in high doses, combined with medications, or taken by vulnerable populations [8–10].

Despite the risks, there is a lack of systematic data on FS use in polymedicated older adults, particularly in community settings. This gap hampers efforts to identify high-risk combinations and implement preventive strategies. The present work aims to (1) describe the patterns of FS use among polymedicated older adults, including type, duration, motivation, and cost; and (2) identify potential FS–drug interactions using validated databases. It is anticipated that the work will provide evidence that informs clinical practice and health policy, supporting safer use of FS in a vulnerable population.

2. Materials and Methods

This cross-sectional study was part of the ESPIEM 2024/2025 cohort under the Healthy Ageing—Egas Moniz Interdisciplinary Project, aimed at promoting rational pharmacotherapy and understanding health behaviors in older adults. A convenience sample of community-dwelling individuals aged 65 or older and on polymedication was recruited by third-year pharmacy students through personal networks. Data were collected via standardized forms and included demographics, medication profile (number/types of chronic medicines), supplement use (product, ingredients, dose, duration, and motivation), and recommendation source (professional advice or self-initiated). Interaction risk was assessed using DrugBank [11] and Medscape Drug Interaction Checker [12] tools to evaluate the potential for supplement–drug interactions based on CYP enzymes and P-glycoprotein pathways. Supplement costs were estimated using reported dosages and market prices to reflect typical monthly expenses. Descriptive statistics were used to summarize supplement use patterns, potential interactions, and associated financial burden.

3. Results and Discussion

Among 98 polymedicated elderly individuals studied, 18 (18.4%) were taking FS, with a total of 21 distinct products reported. These were taken in addition to an average of 4.6 medications. All FS were oral solid dosage forms (mainly tablets and capsules), which did not appear to hinder use despite common dysphagia in the elderly. Women accounted for 66.7% of FS users. The most common indications were musculoskeletal support (43%) and cognitive enhancement (38%). While most supplements (57.2%) were recommended by health professionals, 38.1% were self-initiated (Figure 1). Use was often long-term, with 29% taking FS for 3–6 months and 43% for over 6 months.

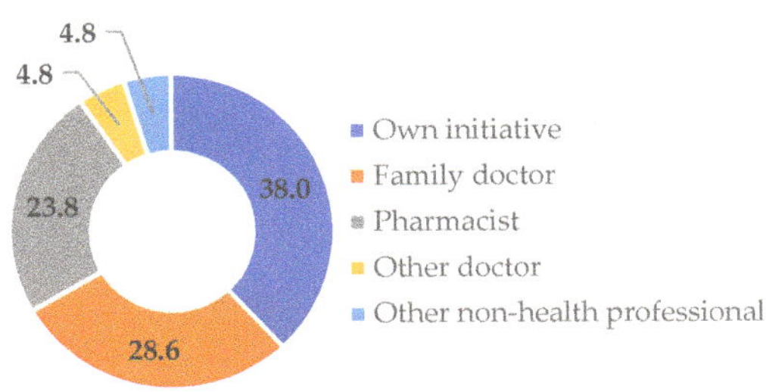

Figure 1. Characterization of the type of prescription or recommendation for FS use (%).

The average monthly supplement cost was €18.23 per patient, reaching up to €55, an added burden for many on limited incomes.

Unlike medicines, FS are less strictly regulated, making their use in polymedicated older adults a concern due to potential clinically relevant interactions and heightened risk of adverse outcomes. In fact, fifteen FS (71%) showed potential CYP/P-gP interactions (Table 1), possibly affecting the metabolism, efficacy, and safety of co-medications. Despite the identification of potential clinically significant interactions, none of these were deemed to represent a life-threatening risk. However, many commonly prescribed drugs, such as statins, proton pump inhibitors, and benzodiazepines, presented interactions, potentially leading to altered efficacy or adverse outcomes. Therefore, clinicians should routinely ask about FS use and consider interactions when taking a medication history. Digital interaction tools and pharmacist-led reviews may enhance safety. Public health strategies should include FS risk education to support safer and more equitable use among older adults.

Table 1. Summary of bioactive constituents in the FS used by study participants (P1–P16), the potential modulatory effects with Cytochrome P450 (CYP) isoenzymes and P-glycoprotein (P-gP), and the concomitant medicines possibly affected [11,12].

P	FS	Bioactive	CYP ↑	CYP ↓	P-gP ↓	Drugs Affected (CYP/Transporter Involved)
1	A	Biotin	1B1	-	No	-
		Lutein	-	2C19	No	Simvastatin; Bromazepam; Pantoprazole (2C19)
		Resveratrol	1A2	1A2; 1A1; 1B1; 3A4; 2D6; 2B6; 2C19; 2C9	No	Betahistine (2D6); Simvastatin (3A4; 2D6; 2C19); Calcitriol (3A4); Acetylsalicylic acid (2C9); Bromazepam (1A2, 2C19; 3A4); Pantoprazole (2C19; 3A4); Spironolactone (3A4)
		Vitamin A	26A1	-	No	-
		Vitamin B1	4B1	-	No	-
		Riboflavin	-	CYP1A2; CYP2C19	No	Simvastatin (2C19); Bromazepam (1A2; 2C19); Pantoprazole (2C19)
		Vitamin B6	-	CYP1A1	No	-
		Vitamin D3	-	CYP1A1; CYP2C8	No	Simvastatin (2C8)
		Vitamin E	3A4	-	No	Simvastatin; Calcitriol; Bromazepam; Pantoprazole; Spironolactone (3A4)
2–4	B	Vitamin D3		1A1; 2C8	No	Atorvastatin (2C8)
5	C	Biotin	1B1	-	No	-
		Niacin	-	2D6; 3A4; 2E1	No	Bisoprolol (3A4; 2D6); Simvastatin (3A4; 2D6); Diazepam (3A4); Budesonide (3A4)
		Vitamin B6	-	1A1	No	-
6	D	DHA	-	2C9	No	-
7	E	Vitamin B6	-	1A1	No	-
		Vitamin D3	-	1A1; 2C8	No	-
8	F	DHA	-	2C9	No	Venlafaxine
		EPA	-	1A2	No	-
		Curcumin	-	3A4; 2C9; 2B6; 1A2; 2D6	Yes	Atorvastatin (3A4/P-gP); Venlafaxine (2D6; 3A4; 2C9/P-gP)
		Piperine	-	3A4	Yes	Atorvastatin (3A4/P-gP); Venlafaxine (3A4/P-gP)
		Vitamin E	3A4	-	No	Atorvastatin; Venlafaxine (3A4)
9	G	Vitamin D3	-	1A1; 2C8	No	Atorvastatin (2C8)
	H	EPA	-	1A2	No	-
		DHA	-	2C9	No	Candesartan (2C9)
10	I	Quercetin	-	2C8; 2D6; 2C9; 1A2; 2E1; 2C19	Yes	Alprazolam (2C9); Bisoprolol (2D6/P-gP)
11	J	DHA	-	2C9	No	Acetylsalicylic acid; Pitavastatin (2C9)
		EPA	-	1A2	No	-
		Vitamin E	3A4	-	No	Pantoprazole; Amlodipine; Silodosin (3A4)

Table 1. *Cont.*

P	FS	Bioactive	CYP ↑	CYP ↓	P-gP ↓	Drugs Affected (CYP/Transporter Involved)
12	K	Vitamin B1	4B1	-	No	-
		Riboflavin	-	1A2; 2C19	No	Esomeprazole (2C19); Simvastatin (2C19); Clozapine (1A2; 2C19); Vortioxetine (2C19)
		Niacin	-	2D6; 3A4; 2E1	No	Clonazepam (3A4); Esomeprazole (3A4); Simvastatin (3A4; 2D6); Clozapine (3A4; 2D6); Betahistine (2D6); Vortioxetine (3A4; 2D6)
		Vitamin B6	-	1A1	No	-
		Biotin	1B1	-	No	-
13	L	Pyridoxine	-	1A1	No	-
14	M	DHA	-	2C9	No	Trimipramine; Valsartan; Rosuvastatin (2C9)
		EPA	-	1A2	No	-
15	N	Niacin	-	2D6; 3A4; 2E1	No	Pantoprazole (3A4); Imatinib (3A4; 2D6)
		Riboflavin	-	1A2; 2C19	No	Pantoprazole (2C19); Imatinib (1A2; 2C19)
16	O	DHA	-	2C9	No	Omeprazole; Fluoxetine (2C9)
		EPA	-	1A2	No	Fluoxetine (1A2)

Interactions are classified based on how FS bioactives affect CYP enzymes and the P-gP transporter involved in drug disposition. Arrows indicate whether these pathways are induced (↑) or inhibited (↓), while "Yes" or "No" under P-gP denotes whether there is a documented transporter inhibition. Lack of interaction (-) means that no current evidence of significant effect exists.

A key limitation of this study is the small number of FS users, which limits statistical power, generalizability, and subgroup (gender, comorbidities, or types of FS used) analysis. The low prevalence may also reflect underreporting, as some participants might not perceive supplements as relevant to their medication regimen or might withhold such information. Additionally, with such a small group of supplement users, the identification of potential supplement–drug interactions is necessarily limited, and clinically significant combinations may not have been captured. These limitations underscore the importance of future studies involving larger and more diverse elderly populations to better characterize supplement use patterns and associated risks in the context of polypharmacy.

4. Conclusions

The use of FS in older adults taking multiple medications reflects vulnerabilities in clinical, financial, and regulatory areas. The findings highlight the need for routine FS screening, the use of interaction tools, and integrated medication review strategies in practice. Public health policies should promote FS literacy and risk awareness, in line with One Health principles for safer ageing.

Author Contributions: M.D.A. and A.I.F. contributed equally to the conceptualization, data acquisition and treatment, writing, illustrating, reviewing, and editing of the manuscript. All authors have read and agreed to the published version of the manuscript.

Funding: This research was funded by Egas Moniz, Cooperativa de Ensino Superior—Envelhecimento Saudável—Projeto Interdisciplinar Egas Moniz (ESPIEM), 2022. M.D.A. and A.I.F. also thank FCT/MCTES for the financial support to CiiEM (10.54499/UIDB/04585/2020) through national funds.

Institutional Review Board Statement: The study was conducted in accordance with the Declaration of Helsinki, and approved by the Ethics Committee of Egas Moniz (file no. 12/30, 25/5/2023).

Informed Consent Statement: Informed consent was obtained from all subjects involved in the study.

Data Availability Statement: The raw data supporting the conclusions of this article will be made available by the authors on request.

Acknowledgments: The authors thank 2024–2025 third-year pharmacy students at Egas Moniz for their assistance with data collection.

Conflicts of Interest: The authors declare no conflicts of interest.

References

1. Maher, R.L.; Hanlon, J.; Hajjar, E.R. Clinical consequences of polypharmacy in elderly. *Expert Opin. Drug Saf.* **2014**, *13*, 57–65. [CrossRef] [PubMed]
2. Morin, L.; Johnell, K.; Laroche, M.-L.; Fastbom, J.; Wastesson, J.W. The epidemiology of polypharmacy in older adults: Register-based prospective cohort study. *Clin. Epidemiol.* **2018**, *10*, 289–298. [CrossRef] [PubMed]
3. Shahverdian, A.; Jafari, M. Dietary supplement safety in older adults: A review of published case reports. *Sr. Care Pharm.* **2025**, *40*, 32–49. [CrossRef] [PubMed]
4. Asher, G.N.; Corbett, A.H.; Hawke, R.L. Common herbal dietary supplement-drug interactions. *Am. Fam. Physician* **2017**, *96*, 101–107. [PubMed]
5. Auxtero, M.D.; Chalante, S.; Abade, M.R.; Jorge, R.; Fernandes, A.I. Potential Herb-Drug Interactions in the Management of Age-Related Cognitive Dysfunction. *Pharmaceutics* **2021**, *13*, 124. [CrossRef] [PubMed]
6. Zhou, S.; Chan, E.; Pan, S.-Q.; Huang, M.; Lee, E.J.D. Pharmacokinetic interactions of drugs with St John's wort. *J. Psychopharmacol.* **2004**, *18*, 262–276. [CrossRef]
7. Izzo, A.A.; Ernst, E. Interactions between herbal medicines and prescribed drugs: An updated systematic review. *Drugs* **2009**, *69*, 1777–1798. [CrossRef] [PubMed]
8. Mazzanti, G.; Menniti-Ippolito, F.; Moro, P.A.; Cassetti, F.; Raschetti, R.; Santuccio, C.; Mastrangelo, S. Hepatotoxicity from green tea: A review of the literature and two unpublished cases. *Eur. J. Clin. Pharmacol.* **2009**, *65*, 331–341. [CrossRef] [PubMed]
9. Teschke, R.; Schwarzenboeck, A.; Hennermann, K.-H. Kava hepatotoxicity: A clinical survey and critical analysis of 26 suspected cases. *Eur. J. Gastroenterol. Hepatol.* **2008**, *20*, 1182–1193. [CrossRef] [PubMed]
10. Bent, S.; Tiedt, T.N.; Odden, M.; Shlipak, M.G. The relative safety of Ephedra compared with other herbal products. *Ann. Intern. Med.* **2003**, *138*, 1006–1007. [CrossRef]
11. DrugBank Online. Available online: https://go.drugbank.com (accessed on 21 May 2025).
12. Drug Interactions Checker-Medscape Drug Reference Database. Available online: https://reference.medscape.com/drug-interactionchecker (accessed on 21 May 2025).

medical sciences forum

Proceeding Paper

Characterisation of the Patient Population Attending the Interstitial Lung Disease Clinic at Hospital Garcia de Orta: Implications for Pulmonary Rehabilitation †

Ana Paula Sequeira [1,2], Ângela Pereira [1,3] and Helena Santa-Clara [4,*]

1 Unidade Funcional de Fisioterapia do Serviço de Medicina Física e Reabilitação, Hospital Garcia de Orta, 2805-267 Almada, Portugal; ana.sequeira@ulsas.min-saude.pt (A.P.S.); angela.pereira@ulsas.min-saude.pt (Â.P.)
2 Departamento de Fisioterapia, Escola Superior de Saúde Atlântica, 2730-036 Oeiras, Portugal
3 Interdisciplinary Research Centre Egas Moniz, Egas Moniz School of Health and Science, 2829-511 Almada, Portugal
4 Centro Interdisciplinar de Estudo da Performance Humana CIPER, Faculdade de Motricidade Humana, Universidade de Lisboa, Cruz Quebrada, 1495-751 Lisboa, Portugal
* Correspondence: santaclara@fmh.ulisboa.pt
† Presented at the 7th CiiEM International Congress 2025—Empowering One Health to Reduce Social Vulnerabilities, Caparica, Portugal, 2–4 July 2025.

Abstract: Interstitial lung diseases (ILDs) are chronic respiratory disorders often leading to dyspnoea, reduced exercise tolerance, and poor quality of life. Pulmonary rehabilitation (PR) improves symptoms and function but remains underused in Portugal, with only ~1% of eligible patients enrolled. This study retrospectively analysed 61 ILD patients at Hospital Garcia de Orta (July–December 2024) to identify PR candidates. Most had idiopathic pulmonary fibrosis (44%), exertional dyspnoea (67.2%), and moderate lung impairment (49%). Comorbidities and risk factors were common. Findings highlight a significant gap between clinical need and access, reinforcing the urgency of structured referral strategies to expand PR availability.

Keywords: interstitial lung disease; pulmonary rehabilitation; idiopathic pulmonary fibrosis; functional impairment; outpatient care

1. Introduction

Interstitial lung diseases (ILDs) comprise a heterogeneous group of conditions characterised by inflammation and/or fibrosis of the pulmonary interstitium, commonly resulting in progressive dyspnoea, exercise intolerance, and a substantial deterioration in quality of life [1–3].

Although pharmacological treatment has advanced in recent years, particularly with the introduction of antifibrotic agents for progressive phenotypes such as idiopathic pulmonary fibrosis (IPF), non-pharmacological approaches, notably pulmonary rehabilitation (PR), remain underutilised [4]. PR is a core component in the management of chronic respiratory diseases. It is cost-effective, safe, and proven to improve dyspnoea, exercise capacity, and health-related quality of life [3,5].

In Portugal, access to PR is extremely limited. Fewer than 1% of patients with chronic obstructive pulmonary disease (COPD), the primary population currently included in PR programmes, are enrolled [6]. Despite robust evidence supporting the efficacy of PR in chronic respiratory diseases, including ILDs [3], its implementation across the country remains inadequate. Existing services are concentrated in large urban hospitals, contributing to disparities in access. Structural, logistical, and awareness-related barriers further hinder effective implementation [6,7].

Additional factors, such as patient scepticism regarding symptomatic improvement and fear of exertion-induced dyspnoea, also limit participation [6]. Furthermore, there is a paucity of local data on the clinical and functional characterisation of ILD patients in specialist outpatient settings, impeding the development of targeted intervention strategies. Defining clinical, functional, and sociodemographic profiles is critical to optimise referral processes and adapt PR programmes to the Portuguese healthcare context, ultimately aiming to enhance outcomes in this population. Community-based and hybrid models emerge as viable strategies to expand coverage, reduce inequities, and improve clinical outcomes in ILDs and other respiratory conditions.

This study aims to characterise the clinical and functional profile of ILD patients followed in the specialised Interstitial Lung Disease Outpatient Clinic at Hospital Garcia de Orta and to identify those eligible for PR referral. The goal is to inform and optimise referral practices and support the implementation of PR programmes within this population.

2. Materials and Methods

This was a retrospective, descriptive study aimed at characterising the clinical and functional profiles of patients followed in the Interstitial Lung Disease Outpatient Clinic of Hospital Garcia de Orta, with the purpose of identifying those who might benefit from pulmonary rehabilitation (PR).

All patients with a confirmed diagnosis of ILD and active follow-up between July and December 2024 were included. Eligibility criteria comprised a documented ILD diagnosis, clinical follow-up within the specified timeframe, and availability of relevant electronic health records.

Data were collected from the electronic clinical record system (SClínico), ensuring anonymity and compliance with the General Data Protection Regulation (GDPR). Extracted data included the following: demographic information (age and sex); clinical ILD diagnosis according to established criteria and coding; symptomatology (dyspnoea on exertion and chronic cough); respiratory functional assessments (spirometry, lung volumes, and diffusing capacity for carbon monoxide—DLCO), when available; risk factors (history of smoking, relevant occupational or environmental exposures); and associated comorbidities, with emphasis on cardiovascular disease, diabetes mellitus, and obstructive sleep apnoea.

The study received approval from the Ethics Committee of Hospital Garcia de Orta on 3 July 2024. All data were anonymised, and no personally identifiable information was collected.

Data analysis was descriptive, using absolute and relative frequencies for categorical variables and mean with standard deviation for continuous variables. Interpretation focused on identifying clinical features consistent with eligibility for PR, including persistent symptoms, pulmonary function impairment, and comorbidities contributing to functional limitation.

3. Results and Discussion

This retrospective study analysed a cohort of 61 ILD patients followed in a specialised clinic between July and December 2024. The cohort had a mean age of 74.7 years, with a slight predominance of females (54%). IPF was the most prevalent diagnosis (44%), followed by other progressive and chronic fibrosing ILDs, consistent with the literature identifying IPF as the most common ILD in elderly populations [3].

Persistent respiratory symptoms, particularly exertional dyspnoea (67.2%) and chronic cough (27.8%), were highly prevalent, indicating frequent functional impairment. Nearly half of the patients had moderate disease severity according to spirometry and DLCO, while 1.6% had severe disease. These findings support the appropriateness of PR, which is recommended for patients with persistent symptoms and functional limitation [6].

Relevant risk factors were identified in 59% of patients, including a history of smoking (40.9%) and environmental/occupational exposures (32.7%), highlighting the influence of external factors in ILD pathogenesis and progression. Common comorbidities included diabetes mellitus (18%), obstructive sleep apnoea (18%), and cardiovascular disease (14.7%), increasing clinical complexity. These findings align with Butler et al. [1], who reported that musculoskeletal, endocrine, and cardiovascular comorbidities were associated with reduced functional gains in PR, underscoring the need for tailored exercise prescriptions.

Notably, 95.1% of patients in this cohort met the clinical criteria for PR referral, and none were referred for PR, revealing a significant mismatch between clinical need and service availability (no PR programme available at HGO). Despite robust evidence demonstrating significant improvements in six-minute walk distance (6MWD) and health-related quality of life with PR [3,8], referral rates remain extremely low in Portugal. Only around 1% of eligible patients are enrolled in structured PR programmes, similar to rates observed in other countries [5].

Evidence also supports improved survival associated with functional gains in the incremental and endurance shuttle walk tests (ISWT and ESWT) among PR participants [9]. Observational studies further suggest reduced five-year mortality in patients demonstrating a positive functional response to PR, although randomised controlled trials are needed to confirm this benefit [10].

Given the high proportion of eligible patients identified in this study, the systematic implementation of clinical screening tools and structured referral pathways in ILD clinics is essential. Regular assessment of dyspnoea, pulmonary function, and exercise capacity would enable early identification of PR candidates and promote equitable access to this beneficial intervention.

Limitations of this study include its retrospective design based on electronic health records, with no objective functional testing such as the 6MWD. The single-centre and small sample size also limit the generalisability of findings. Nevertheless, the results provide a realistic overview of clinical practice in a specialised centre and highlight the urgent need to expand access to PR as a core component of ILD management.

4. Conclusions

In this cohort, a substantial proportion of ILD patients met clinical criteria for referral to pulmonary rehabilitation. Recent evidence confirms that PR improves functional capacity, reduces symptoms, and enhances quality of life, with possible survival benefits [11].

However, access to this intervention remains critically limited in Portugal. The following measures are recommended: systematic integration of PR screening into ILD clinics; development of structured referral pathways; implementation of alternative models such as home-based or hybrid programmes with remote supervision; and ongoing training and awareness initiatives targeting both healthcare professionals and patients.

Adopting these strategies, in line with international best practices, may increase referral rates and improve clinical outcomes and quality of life for this vulnerable population [12,13].

Author Contributions: Conceptualization, A.P.S. and Â.P.; methodology, A.P.S.; software, A.P.S.; validation, A.P.S., Â.P. and H.S.-C.; formal analysis, A.P.S.; investigation, A.P.S.; resources, A.P.S.; data curation, A.P.S.; writing—original draft preparation, A.P.S.; writing—review and editing Â.P. and H.S.-C.; visualization A.P.S.; supervision, Â.P. and H.S.-C.; project administration, A.P.S. All authors have read and agreed to the published version of the manuscript.

Funding: This research received no external funding.

Institutional Review Board Statement: The study was conducted in accordance with the Declaration of Helsinki and approved by the Ethics Committee of Hospital Garcia de Orta (3 July 2024).

Informed Consent Statement: Informed consent was obtained from all subjects involved in the study.

Data Availability Statement: The datasets presented in this article are not readily available because privacy restrictions.

Acknowledgments: We acknowledge the support given by Miguel Lopes (Director of Pneumology) and Susana Farinha (Director of Physical Medicine and Rehabilitation) by allowing access to the population and registration.

Conflicts of Interest: The authors declare no conflicts of interest.

References

1. Butler, S.J.; Li, L.S.K.; Ellerton, L.; Gershon, A.S.; Goldstein, R.S.; Brooks, D. Prevalence of comorbidities and impact on pulmonary rehabilitation outcomes. *ERJ Open Res.* **2019**, *5*, 00264–2019. [CrossRef] [PubMed]
2. Cottin, V.; Hirani, N.A.; Hotchkin, D.L.; Nambiar, A.M.; Ogura, T.; Otaola, M.; Skowasch, D.; Park, J.S.; Poonyagariyagorn, H.K.; Wuyts, W.; et al. Presentation, diagnosis and clinical course of the spectrum of progressive-fibrosing interstitial lung diseases. *Eur. Respir. Rev.* **2018**, *27*, 180076. [CrossRef] [PubMed]
3. Dowman, L.; Hill, C.J.; May, A.; Holland, A.E. Pulmonary rehabilitation for interstitial lung disease. *Cochrane Database Syst. Rev.* **2021**, *2*, CD006322. [CrossRef] [PubMed]
4. George, P.M.; Wells, A.U.; Jenkins, R.G. Pulmonary fibrosis and COVID-19: The potential role for antifibrotic therapy. *Lancet Respir. Med.* **2020**, *8*, 807–815. [CrossRef] [PubMed]
5. Menson, K.E.; Dowman, L. Pulmonary Rehabilitation for Diseases Other Than COPD. *J. Cardiopulm. Rehabil. Prev.* **2024**, *44*, 425–431. [CrossRef] [PubMed]
6. Silva, L.; Mota, Â.; Lemos, L.; Santos, M.; Cunha, H.; Maricoto, T.; Costa, P.; Padilha, M. Characterisation of Patients with Chronic Obstructive Pulmonary Disease (COPD) From an Urban Municipality in the Northern Region of Portugal: A Cross-Sectional Study. *Cureus* **2024**, *16*, e59262. [CrossRef] [PubMed]
7. Sociedade Portuguesa de Pneumologia. *Reabilitação Respiratória: Documento de Consenso*; SPP: Lisbon, Portugal, 2021.
8. Spruit, M.A.; Singh, S.J.; Garvey, C.; ZuWallack, R.; Nici, L.; Rochester, C.; Hill, K.; Holland, A.E.; Lareau, S.C.; Man, W.D.-C.; et al. An official American Thoracic Society/European Respiratory Society statement: Key concepts and advances in pulmonary rehabilitation. *Am. J. Respir. Crit. Care Med.* **2013**, *188*, e13–e64. [CrossRef] [PubMed]
9. Zatloukal, J.; Houchen-Wolloff, L.; Ward, S.; Khan, F.; Singh, S.J. Minimum important difference of shuttle walk tests in patients with interstitial lung disease following pulmonary rehabilitation. *ERJ Open Res.* **2025**, *11*, 00601–2024. [CrossRef]
10. Gushken, F.; Degani-Costa, L.H.; Colognese, T.C.P.; Rodrigues, M.T.; Zanetti, M.; Bonamigo-Filho, J.L.; de Matos, L.D.N.J. Barriers to enrollment in pulmonary rehabilitation: Medical knowledge analysis. *Einstein* **2021**, *19*, eAO6115. [CrossRef] [PubMed]
11. Hoffman, M.; Mellerick, C.; Symons, K.; Glaspole, I.; Holland, A. Pulmonary rehabilitation for interstitial lung disease: Referral and patient experiences. *Chronic Respir. Dis.* **2021**, *18*, 14799731211046022. [CrossRef]
12. Holland, A. Physiotherapy management of interstitial lung disease. *J. Physiother.* **2022**, *68*, 158–164. [CrossRef] [PubMed]
13. Molgat-Seon, Y.; Schaeffer, M.; Ryerson, C.; Guenette, J. Exercise Pathophysiology in Interstitial Lung Disease. *Clin. Chest Med.* **2019**, *40*, 405–420. [CrossRef] [PubMed]

medical sciences forum

MDPI

Proceeding Paper

Determinants of Exclusive Breastfeeding Duration: A Population-Based Study from Southern Portugal †

Flávia Oliveira [1,2,*] and Sónia Vicente [3]

1 Unidade Local de Saúde do Algarve E.P.E., 8000-386 Faro, Portugal
2 Alcoitão School of Health Sciences, 2649-506 Alcabideche, Portugal
3 Egas Moniz Center for Interdisciplinary Research (CiiEM), Egas Moniz School of Health & Science, Caparica, 2829-511 Almada, Portugal; svicente@egasmoniz.edu.pt
* Correspondence: foliveira@ulsalg.min-saude.pt
† Presented at the 7th CiiEM International Congress 2025—Empowering One Health to Reduce Social Vulnerabilities, Caparica, Portugal, 2–4 July 2025.

Abstract: Exclusive breastfeeding for the first six months is the gold standard in infant nutrition, yet rates in Europe remain below recommendations. This descriptive cross-sectional study identified maternal, perinatal and social determinants associated with shorter exclusive breastfeeding duration in the Algarve region. Statistically significant factors included in-hospital formula use, caesarean section, lack of skin-to-skin contact, and negative or absent previous experience of breastfeeding. In-hospital formula use and previous breastfeeding duration emerged as key predictors. These findings emphasise the importance of integrated strategies across the healthcare, workplace, and policy sectors, aligned with the lived experiences of women, to effectively support breastfeeding.

Keywords: exclusive breastfeeding; breastfeeding duration; breastfeeding support; maternal determinants; southern Portugal

1. Introduction

Breast milk is a unique living food [1] that adapts to each baby's needs, providing complete nutrition for the first six months [2–4]. Exclusive breastfeeding (EBF) during this period is the global public health standard due to its proven benefits [5].

In the 20th century, breastfeeding (BF) rates declined, especially in industrialised countries [6], leading to global strategies such as the Global Breastfeeding Collective (GBC) [4]. Despite this, global BF rates remain below World Health Organization (WHO) and GBC targets [5,7], with several factors linked to shorter EBF duration [4,8–12]. Europe has the lowest rates of all WHO regions [13,14].

In Portugal, there is no published data on BF and its determinants in the Algarve region. This study aimed to determine the prevalence of and the factors influencing BF during the first six months of life in the Algarve region.

2. Materials and Methods

An observational, descriptive, and cross-sectional study is presented.

2.1. Participants and Recruitment

A total of 464 mothers of infants aged 6–24 months, residing in the Algarve, participated in the study. Inclusion criteria were literacy in Portuguese and informed consent. Medical contraindications to breastfeeding served as exclusion criteria.

Sample size was based on 5869 children registered at Algarve health centres, born between 1 July 2021 and 31 December 2022, with a 5% sampling error and 95% confidence level. Recruitment occurred via social media, day care and health centres, and maternal and child health professionals. Participation was voluntary and anonymous.

2.2. Data Collection

Data was collected between 1 July and 30 September 2023. A self-administered pretested online questionnaire was designed based on guidelines and the work of Caldeira et al. [15], and validated by a Delphi panel. The final questionnaire comprised 44 questions, all mandatory to prevent missing data.

2.3. Data Analysis

Data were analysed using SPSS v28.0. Independent sample t-tests assessed associations between EBF duration and parity, prenatal BF sessions, previous BF experience, formula use in hospital, skin-to-skin contact, smoking, partner support, and maternal education. Education level was recoded as primary/secondary vs. higher. Effect size was calculated using Cohen's d. Pearson's correlation assessed associations between EBF duration, maternal age, and prior BF duration. Welch's ANOVA tested the effect of birth type on EBF duration, with eta-squared as effect size and Games–Howell for post hoc comparisons. A multiple regression identified predictors of EBF duration. A p-value of <0.05 was considered significant.

3. Results

Of 503 responses, 464 were eligible (age 18–49, M = 33.99). Most had a partner (97.4%), were primiparous (55.2%), had high education (60.34%), received BF information during pregnancy (79.1%), and only 27.2% stayed home $\geq$6 months. Full-term births occurred in 95.3%, where 44.4% were caesarean. In the hospital, 85.3% of mothers initiated breastfeeding within the first hour after birth, 45.3% of infants were given formula (mainly via cup or bottle), and 76.9% experienced immediate skin-to-skin contact, with 43.9% lasting less than one hour. At discharge, 73.1% were EBF and common challenges reported during the first weeks included cracked nipples. (53.2%), pain (44%), and latch difficulties (28.4%). Family support was reported by 68.1%, especially from partners (87.9%). Reasons for stopping BF included perceived insufficient milk (31.2%), and latch issues (18.6%). Among multiparous women, 40.5% had prior BF experiences and 81.9% considered it positive. BF and EBF rates declined over time: at 15 days, 94% BF and 78.9% EBF; at 3 months, 85.1% and 69%; at 6 months, 74.4% and 38.1%.

Statistical analysis showed the following: small effect for parity [t = 2.213, p = 0.027, d = 0.205], prenatal BF sessions [t = 2.089, p = 0.038, d = 0.209], prior BF experience [t = 2.555, p = 0.011, d = 0.237], education [t = 2.558, p = 0.011, d = 0.243], duration of previous BF [R = 0.269, $p \leq 0.01$], moderate effects for quality (positive/negative) of prior BF [t = 3.290, $p < 0.001$, d = 0.679], skin-to-skin contact [t = 3.811, $p < 0.001$, d = 0.449], and large effect for use of formula in hospital [t = −9.698, $p < 0.001$, d = 0.938]. Vaginal births were associated with longer EBF than caesarean [Mean Difference = 32.57, $p < 0.001$] [Fw (2, 149.746) = 10.040, $p < 0.001$, $\eta^2 = 0.043$]. Multiple regression identified formula use in hospital (Beta = 0.373, $p < 0.001$) and previous BF duration (Beta = 0.213, p = 0.002) as significant predictors. No significant associations were found for age, smoking, or partner support.

4. Discussion

The study's findings of 38.1% EBF rate at six months is significantly below the GBC 2030 target. This decline from 59.5% at five months may be linked to shorter parental leave

(72.8% of the sample) and early complementary feeding due to childcare arrangements. The current paid parental leave policy in Portugal may pose a barrier to the EBF continuation for six months. Additionally, inadequate workplace support contributes to early formula introduction [4]. Although the WHO recommends six months of EBF, the European Society for Paediatric Gastroenterology, Hepatology, and Nutrition suggests introducing complementary feeding between four and six months [16], leading to inconsistent advice that may impact EBF duration.

Caesareans (44.4%) were linked to shorter EBF duration, reduced early skin-to-skin contact, and delayed BF initiation. Nearly half of caesarean mothers missed early contact, which contributed to missed early BF opportunities. Only 42.8% had skin-to-skin contact lasting at least one hour, despite its known benefits [17].

In-hospital formula use, found in 45.3% of infants, was associated with shorter EBF duration, likely influenced by high caesarean rates and staff limitations. The WHO and UNICEF stress that formula should only be introduced when necessary, yet early supplementation disrupts BF [18], potentially causing nipple trauma, pain, and latch issues in 53.2%, 44%, and 28.4% of mothers, respectively. Limited postnatal support, reported by only 34.5% of mothers, may exacerbate these challenges.

Nearly half of participants (49.8%) had ceased BF, with the primary reason being perceived insufficient milk, echoing national trends [19]. This highlights the need for better support and education to address misconceptions about milk supply.

Frequency of BF sessions during pregnancy was positively associated with longer EBF duration. This education helps women manage challenges in the early and later stages of BF. Family-centred interventions, targeting both mothers and partners, are essential for overcoming social and environmental barriers to BF [4,8,20].

Although partner support was not significantly associated with EBF duration, the literature suggests that active involvement enhances BF success [6,21]. Despite 87.9% reporting partner support, variations in perceived support may explain the lack of significance. Further research on partner roles, especially in same-gender partnerships, is needed to refine intervention strategies.

Prior BF experience positively influenced subsequent EBF, confirming the study's findings. Experienced mothers often exhibit greater confidence and motivation to continue BF, while inexperienced mothers are more affected by sociocultural factors [10].

Convenience sampling limits representativeness and recall bias is possible due to retrospective questions. To minimise bias, the questionnaire was kept concise and focused on relevant items.

5. Conclusions

The study highlights that parental leave, hospital practices, and maternal perceptions significantly impact breastfeeding outcomes. The six month EBF rate remains below WHO targets, reflecting national trends. Improving outcomes requires stronger institutional support, better healthcare training, more baby-friendly facilities, community breastfeeding spaces, and increased public awareness. Aligning policies with mothers' real-life experiences is key to fostering supportive environments for breastfeeding.

Author Contributions: Conceptualization: F.O. and S.V.; data curation: F.O.; formal analysis: F.O.; investigation: F.O.; methodology: F.O. and S.V.; writing—original draft preparation: F.O.; supervision: S.V.; writing—review and editing: S.V. All authors have read and agreed to the published version of the manuscript.

Funding: This research received no external funding.

Institutional Review Board Statement: The study was conducted in accordance with the Declaration of Helsinki and approved by the Health Ethics Committee and the Board of Directors of the Regional Health Administration of Algarve (ARS Algarve), I.P (June 2023).

Informed Consent Statement: Informed consent was obtained from all subjects involved in the study.

Data Availability Statement: The raw data supporting the conclusions of this article will be made available by the authors on request.

Conflicts of Interest: The authors declare no conflicts of interest.

Abbreviations

The following abbreviations are used in this manuscript:

EBF	Exclusive breastfeeding
BF	Breastfeeding
WHO	World Health Organization
GBC	Global Breastfeeding Collective

References

1. González, H.F.; Carosella, M.; Fernández, A. Nutritional Risks among Not Exclusively Breastfed Infants in the First 6 Months of Life. *Arch. Argent. Pediatr.* **2021**, *119*, E582–E588. [CrossRef] [PubMed]
2. Hernández-Cordero, S.; Pérez-Escamilla, R. What will It Take to Increase Breastfeeding? *Matern. Child Nutr.* **2022**, *18*, e13371. [CrossRef] [PubMed]
3. Christian, P.; Smith, E.R.; Lee, S.E.; Vargas, A.J.; Bremer, A.A.; Raiten, D.J. The Need to Study Human Milk as a Biological System. *Am. J. Clin. Nutr.* **2021**, *113*, 1063–1072. [CrossRef] [PubMed]
4. Patil, D.S.; Pundir, P.; Dhyani, V.S.; Krishnan, J.B.; Parsekar, S.S.; D'Souza, S.M.; Ravishankar, N.; Renjith, V. A Mixed-Methods Systematic Review on Barriers to Exclusive Breastfeeding. *Nutr. Health* **2020**, *26*, 323–346. [CrossRef] [PubMed]
5. Amoo, T.B.; Popoola, T.; Lucas, R. Promoting the Practice of Exclusive Breastfeeding: A Philosophic Scoping Review. *BMC Pregnancy Childbirth* **2022**, *22*, 380. [CrossRef] [PubMed]
6. Prentice, A.M. Breastfeeding in the Modern World. *Ann. Nutr. Metab.* **2022**, *78*, 29–38. [CrossRef] [PubMed]
7. Alayón, S.; Varela, V.; Mukuria-Ashe, A.; Alvey, J.; Milner, E.; Pedersen, S.; Yourkavitch, J. Exclusive Breastfeeding: Measurement to Match the Global Recommendation. *Matern. Child Nutr.* **2022**, *18*, e13409. [CrossRef]
8. Cohen, S.; Alexander, D.; Krebs, N.; Young, B.; Cabana, M.; Erdmann, P.; Hays, N.; Bezold, C.; Levin-Sparenberg, E.; Turini, M.; et al. Factors Associated with Breastfeeding Initiation and Continuation: A Meta-Analysis. *J. Pediatr.* **2018**, *203*, 190–196.e21. [CrossRef]
9. Wu, Q.; Tang, N.; Wacharasin, C. Factors Influencing Exclusive Breastfeeding for 6 Months Postpartum: A Systematic Review. *Int. J. Nurs. Knowl.* **2022**, *33*, 290–303. [CrossRef] [PubMed]
10. Huang, Y.; Ouyang, Y.; Redding, S.R. Previous Breastfeeding Experience and Its Influence on Breastfeeding Outcomes in Subsequent Births: A Systematic Review. *Women Birth* **2019**, *32*, 303–309. [CrossRef] [PubMed]
11. Pérez-Escamilla, R.; Hromi-Fiedler, A.; Rhodes, E.C.; Neves, P.A.R.; Vaz, J.; Vilar-Compte, M.; Segura-Pérez, S.; Nyhan, K. Impact of Prelacteal Feeds and Neonatal Introduction of Breast Milk Substitutes on Breastfeeding Outcomes: A Systematic Review and Meta Analysis. *Matern. Child Nutr.* **2022**, *18*, e13368. [CrossRef] [PubMed]
12. Kehinde, J.; O'Donnell, C.; Grealish, A. The Effectiveness of Prenatal Breastfeeding Education on Breastfeeding Uptake Postpartum: A Systematic Review. *Midwifery* **2023**, *118*, 103579. [CrossRef]
13. Zakarija-Grković, I.; Cattaneo, A.; Bettinelli, M.E.; Pilato, C.; Vassallo, C.; Borg Buontempo, M.; Gray, H.; Meynell, C.; Wise, P.; Harutyunyan, S.; et al. Are Our Babies off to a Healthy Start? The State of Implementation of the Global Strategy for Infant and Young Child Feeding in Europe. *Int. Breastfeed. J.* **2020**, *15*, 51. [CrossRef] [PubMed]
14. Theurich, M.A.; Davanzo, R.; Busck-Rasmussen, M.; Díaz-Gómez, N.M.; Brennan, C.; Kylberg, E.; Bærug, A.; McHugh, L.; Weikert, C.; Abraham, K.; et al. Breastfeeding Rates and Programs in Europe: A Survey of 11 National Breastfeeding Committees and Representatives. *J. Pediatr. Gastroenterol. Nutr.* **2019**, *68*, 400–407. [CrossRef] [PubMed]
15. Caldeira, T.; Moreira, P.; Pinto, E. Aleitamento Materno: Estudo Dos Factores Relacionados Com o Seu Abandono. *Rev. Port. Clínica Geral* **2007**, *23*, 685–699. [CrossRef]
16. Fewtrell, M.; Bronsky, J.; Campoy, C.; Domellof, M.; Embleton, N.; Mis, N.; Hojsak, I.; Hulst, J.; Indrio, F.; Lapillonne, A.; et al. Complementary Feeding: A Position Paper by the European Society for Paediatric Gastroenterology, Hepatology, and Nutrition (ESPGHAN) Committee on Nutrition. *J. Pediatr. Gastroenterol. Nutr.* **2017**, *64*, 119–132. [CrossRef]

17. Brimdyr, K.; Stevens, J.; Svensson, K.; Blair, A.; Maffei, C.T.-; Grady, J.; Bastarache, L.; Crenshaw, J.T.; Regina, E.; Giugliani, J.; et al. Skin-to-Skin Contact after Birth: Developing a Research and Practice Guideline. *Acta Paediatr. Int. J. Paediatr.* **2023**, *112*, 1633–1643. [CrossRef] [PubMed]
18. WHO; UNICEF. *Implementation Guidance: Protecting, Promoting and Supporting Breastfeeding in Facilities Providing Maternity and Newborn Services—The Revised Baby-Friendly Hospital Initiative*; WHO: Geneva, Switzerland, 2018.
19. Lanzaro, C.; Santos, P.; Guerra, A.; Hespanhol, A.P.; Esteves, M.J. Prevalência Do Aleitamento Materno: Comparação Entre Uma População Urbana e Uma População Rural No Norte de Portugal. *Acta Pediátrica Port.* **2015**, *46*, 101–108.
20. Gao, H.; Wang, J.; An, J.; Liu, S.; Li, Y.; Ding, S.; Zhang, Y.; Chen, Y. Effects of Prenatal Professional Breastfeeding Education for the Family. *Sci. Rep.* **2022**, *12*, 10–13. [CrossRef] [PubMed]
21. Koksal, I.; Acikgoz, A.; Cakirli, M. The Effect of a Father's Support on Breastfeeding: A Systematic Review. *Breastfeed. Med.* **2022**, *17*, 711–722. [CrossRef] [PubMed]

medical sciences forum

MDPI

Proceeding Paper

Behind the Behaviour: Supporting Young Offenders Through Forensic Psychology †

Iris Almeida [1,2,*], Ana Francisca Matos [1], Diana Pais [1] and Carolina Nobre [2]

[1] Egas Moniz Center for Interdisciplinary Research (CiiEM), Egas Moniz School of Health & Science, Caparica, 2829-511 Almada, Portugal; anafranciscamms@outlook.com (A.F.M.); didimcp01@gmail.com (D.P.)

[2] Gabinete de Informação e Atendimento à Vítima: Espaço Cidadania e Justiça (GIAV), DIAP Regional de Lisboa, Campus de Justiça, Avenida D. João II, Edifício E, 1990-097 Lisbon, Portugal; carolinanobrepsic@gmail.com

* Correspondence: ialmeida@egasmoniz.edu.pt

† Presented at the 7th CiiEM International Congress 2025—Empowering One Health to Reduce Social Vulnerabilities, Caparica, Portugal, 2–4 July 2025.

Abstract: This study highlights the role of forensic psychology in supporting juvenile offenders within the Portuguese Justice System. Forensic psychologists ensure that legal proceedings are developmentally appropriate and psychologically informed, helping minors to understand and participate in the process. Data from the Victims Information and Assistance Office (GIAV) show that, between 2020 and 2025, 87 juvenile offenders (54 boys and 33 girls) were supported, with theft and drug trafficking being the most common crimes. Girls were more often involved in theft, and boys were more often involved in drug trafficking. Forensic psychology adds critical value by promoting rehabilitation, safeguarding rights, and contributing to fair, proportionate, and context-sensitive decisions.

Keywords: young offenders; forensic psychology; Portuguese justice system

1. Introduction

Forensic psychology plays a crucial role in supporting juvenile offenders throughout legal proceedings by providing a developmental, contextualised, and evidence-based understanding of their behaviours. In the Portuguese Justice System, the involvement of forensic psychologists in juvenile cases—particularly those involving young offenders under the Law on the Protection of Children and Young People in Danger and the Educational Guardianship Law [1]—is essential to ensure that responses to offending behaviour are fair, proportionate, and informed by the psychological characteristics and life contexts of the minors involved. Forensic psychologists contribute at multiple procedural stages, including police interviews, judicial hearings, and pre-sentencing assessments. Their presence ensures that the minor comprehends the nature and implications of the proceedings and is supported in providing their account in a developmentally appropriate and psychologically safe manner. This is particularly important to avoid secondary victimisation and to uphold the procedural rights of minors, in line with both national legislation and international standards—such as Directive (EU) 2016/800 on procedural safeguards for children and the UN Convention on the Rights of the Child [2,3]. In Portugal, psychologists working with juvenile offenders often form part of multidisciplinary teams operating in child protection commissions (CPCJ), juvenile courts, and detention centers. Within these contexts, forensic psychologists conduct comprehensive psychosocial assessments and collaborate on the development and monitoring of individualised educational plans. These plans not only address legal requirements but are designed to promote the juvenile's reintegration into society, their psychosocial rehabilitation, and the construction of prosocial life projects.

Furthermore, forensic psychologists advise judicial authorities on the minor's maturity, psychological functioning, trauma history, family context, and capacity for change. This information is vital in ensuring that judicial decisions regarding educational measures—such as community-based monitoring or custodial placement—are appropriate and proportionate to both the offence and the developmental profile of the juvenile.

During the execution phase of court-imposed measures, psychologists remain involved through ongoing support, regular re-assessment, and progress reporting to the judiciary. In custodial settings, they also contribute to the design and implementation of therapeutic interventions, including mental health care and emotional regulation programmes, increasingly recognised as essential for young offenders presenting with psychiatric comorbidities or substance misuse issues.

Finally, forensic psychologists act as a bridge between the justice system and the welfare system, especially in cases where young people are simultaneously in conflict with the law and in need of protective measures. Their expertise allows for nuanced case formulations that distinguish between risk and vulnerability, and that advocate for integrated responses across the child protection, education, and criminal justice sectors.

Therefore, the purpose of this study is to explore and illustrate the essential functions of forensic psychology in supporting juvenile offenders within legal proceedings, and to highlight the added value of evidence-informed developmental approaches in promoting fair justice and sustainable rehabilitation.

2. Methods

Based within the Victims' Information and Assistance Office (GIAV), within the Public Prosecutor's Office, the forensic psychologists provided support to 87 juvenile offenders [54 boys (62%) and 33 girls (38%)], aged between 15 and 17 years old (M = 16.7, SD = 0.55), throughout the years 2020 to 2025. The forensic psychologists at GIAV accompanied juvenile offenders to several legal proceedings, namely constitution of the defendant (n = 58, 67%) and provisional suspension of proceedings (n = 19, 22%). Nonetheless, other interventions (e.g., first judicial interrogation and trial) are also part of GIAV's scope of work (n = 10, 11%).

Data were collected from GIAV's database.

3. Results and Discussion

Regarding the crimes committed, the results show that 26 (30%) juvenile offenders were involved in theft, 17 (20%) in drug trafficking, and 10 (11%) in unlicensed driving, as well as involvement in other crimes, for instance, physical assault and illegal possession of a firearm (n = 34, 39%) (Table 1).

Table 1. Results regarding the most prevalent criminal offences.

Criminal Offence	n	%
Theft	26	30
Drug trafficking	17	20
Unlicensed driving	10	11
Others (e.g., physical assault, illegal possession of a firearm)	34	39

Furthermore, they indicate that girls are more frequently associated with theft (twenty-three girls and three boys), while boys are more often linked to drug trafficking (sixteen boys and one girl) (Table 2).

Table 2. Cross-checking data with gender.

Criminal Offence	Female	Male
Theft	23	3
Drug trafficking	1	16
Unlicensed driving	1	9
Others (e.g., physical assault, illegal possession of a firearm)	5	29

These findings are corroborated by literature (e.g., [4,5]) and can reflect broader social, economic, and possibly cultural dynamics that shape the pathways into delinquency for each gender. Compared to other crimes, theft is more common among girls as it is frequently motivated by peer pressure, a desire for prestige items, or a coping strategy for emotional pain or unfulfilled monetary requirements [5]. Additionally, it is seen to be a low-risk, low-violence crime, which might help to explain why theft, for instance, shoplifting, is so common among females as they are less likely to engage in aggressive or confrontational criminal activity [5]. On the other hand, the second most common offence in this study, drug trafficking, is primarily linked to boys. This is consistent with prior research showing that male juveniles tend to engage in organised or group-based illegal activity, which is frequently connected to early criminal socialisation, exposure to street networks, and masculinity norms [6].

These gendered delinquency trends highlight the importance of developing tailored intervention approaches [6,7]. To achieve this, an in-depth understanding of the underlying motives and contextual factors behind offences such as shoplifting is essential. Such an understanding can inform the design of gender-sensitive prevention and rehabilitation programmes that directly address the psychological and social vulnerabilities contributing to these minors' involvement in delinquent behaviour [6,7]. Ultimately, this approach aims not only to intervene effectively but also to reduce the recurrence and escalation of such behaviours [7].

4. Conclusions

Forensic psychology is a pivotal component of the juvenile justice system, translating psychological science into judicial practice to deliver decisions that are developmentally informed, fair, and tailored to the unique needs of each young offender [6,7]. The experience at GIAV exemplifies how embedding forensic psychologists throughout all the procedural phases—from initial hearings to the execution of measures—enhances the justice system's capacity to interpret offending behaviours within their broader psychosocial contexts, resulting in more nuanced, individualised, and just outcomes.

The distinct gender-related offending patterns observed underscore an urgent need for gender-responsive evidence-based intervention strategies. Programmes targeting girls should prioritise addressing emotional coping mechanisms, peer influences, and socio-economic vulnerabilities linked to offences such as theft, while interventions for boys must confront the influence of group dynamics, street socialisation, and masculinity norms prevalent in drug trafficking [5–7]. Such targeted approaches have the potential not only to improve rehabilitation effectiveness but also to significantly reduce rates of recidivism and support more positive social reintegration.

From a policy standpoint, this study advocates for the formal institutionalisation of forensic psychologists within every stage of juvenile justice procedures, thereby safeguarding minors' procedural rights and ensuring that decisions are underpinned by robust empirical evidence and developmental insight (cf. Directive (EU) 2016/800 [2]). Achieving this requires dedicated investment in specialist training, resource allocation, and the development of multidisciplinary teams equipped to address the complex needs of juvenile offenders comprehensively.

Academically, the study contributes meaningful empirical evidence to the growing literature supporting rehabilitative, developmental, and evidence-based approaches in juvenile justice [6,7]. It emphasises the critical role of detailed psychological assessments that differentiate risk from vulnerability, thereby guiding judicial decision-making towards more ethical and effective outcomes. Furthermore, it highlights areas for future research, particularly regarding the long-term impacts of tailored interventions and the influence of sociocultural factors specific to the Portuguese context.

In summary, forensic psychology not only protects the rights of children and young people in conflict with the law but also drives systemic transformation towards a justice system that is inclusive, equitable, and prioritises sustainable rehabilitation. This dual role ultimately promotes healthier outcomes for individuals and contributes to broader societal wellbeing [3,6,7].

Author Contributions: Conceptualisation, I.A.; methodology, I.A., D.P. and A.F.M.; formal analysis, I.A., A.F.M. and D.P.; writing—original draft preparation, I.A.; writing—review and editing, I.A., A.F.M. and D.P.; visualisation, C.N.; supervision, C.N. and I.A. All authors have read and agreed to the published version of the manuscript.

Funding: This research received no external funding.

Institutional Review Board Statement: This study is part of a protocol established among the Portuguese Public Prosecutor's Office and Egas Moniz School of Health & Science to assess and analyse the characteristics of offenders in the field of violence. The strictness of ethical and deontological principles is safeguarded once criminal records have restricted access by law (including judicial secrecy), all ethical standards of scientific research were respected, as well as the Code of Ethics of the Order of Portuguese Psychologists and the General Data Protection Regulation.Therefore, all assessed subjects gave their informed consent, and their data were processed anonymously. This study was conducted in accordance with the Declaration of Helsinki, and the protocol was approved by the Ethics Committee of Egas Moniz School of Health & Science—One Justice Project: The Forensic Psychology in Justice and Community (number 1231/23—29 June 2023).

Informed Consent Statement: Informed consent for participation was obtained from all subjects involved in the study.

Data Availability Statement: The datasets presented in this article are not readily available because part of information derives from criminal records.

Conflicts of Interest: The authors declare no conflicts of interest.

References

1. European e-Justice Portal. Rights of Minors in Court Proceedings. 2024. Available online: https://e-justice.europa.eu/topics/your-rights/rights-minors-court-proceedings_en (accessed on 16 June 2025).
2. United Nations Convention on the Rights of the Child [UNCRC]. *Convention on the Rights of the Child*; UNCRC: Geneva, Switzerland, 1989; Available online: https://www.unicef.org/child-rights-convention/convention-text (accessed on 16 June 2025).
3. Council of Europe. *Guidelines of the Committee of Ministers of the Council of Europe on Child-Friendly Justice*; Council of Europe: London, UK, 2010; Available online: https://www.coe.int/en/web/children/child-friendly-justice (accessed on 16 June 2025).
4. Campaniello, N. *Women in Crime*; IZA World of Labor: Bonn, Germany, 2014; p. 105. Available online: https://www.econstor.eu/bitstream/10419/125333/1/iza-wol-105.pdf (accessed on 16 June 2025).

5. Caputo, G.; King, A. Shoplifting: Work, agency, and gender. *Fem. Criminol.* **2011**, *6*, 159–177. [CrossRef]
6. Marshall, H. *Young Men's Perspectives on Child Criminal Exploitation and Their Involvement in County Lines Drug Dealing: An Intersectional Analysis*; Policy Press eBooks: Bristol, UK, 2022; pp. 87–101. [CrossRef]
7. Miller, S.; Winn, D.; Taylor, J.; Wiki, T. *Girls' Relational Orientation and Interpersonal Dynamics of Delinquency*; Springer eBooks: Berlin/Heidelberg, Germany, 2011; pp. 85–101.

medical sciences forum

MDPI

Proceeding Paper

Legitimising Beliefs About Intimate Partner Violence: Insights from Portuguese Forensic Cases †

Iris Almeida *, Guilherme Sena, Maria Beatriz Ribeiro and Ricardo Ventura Baúto

Laboratory of Forensic and Psychological Sciences Egas Moniz, CiiEM—Egas Moniz Center for Interdisciplinary Research, Egas Moniz School of Health & Science, Caparica, 2829-511 Almada, Portugal; guisenacosta@gmail.com (G.S.); tiz2001@gmail.com (M.B.R.); rbauto@egasmoniz.edu.pt (R.V.B.)

* Correspondence: ialmeida@egasmoniz.edu.pt

† Presented at the 7th CiiEM International Congress 2025—Empowering One Health to Reduce Social Vulnerabilities, Caparica, Portugal, 2–4 July 2025.

Abstract: This study explores legitimising beliefs about intimate partner violence (IPV) among Portuguese forensic cases. Using the ECVC scale, data from 45 assessed individuals revealed that IPV offenders—particularly men, those with lower education levels, and certain occupational groups—endorse beliefs that justify, minimise, or excuse violence. The most prevalent were trivialising minor violence and protecting family privacy. These findings align with the literature on the influence of patriarchal norms and social inequalities in sustaining IPV. These results highlight the importance of addressing underlying gender ideologies in prevention and intervention efforts, especially in forensic and justice-related psychological practice.

Keywords: intimate partner violence; beliefs; forensic cases

1. Introduction

Intimate partner violence (IPV) is a pervasive public health issue with significant psychological and social consequences [1]. Exposure to IPV is strongly associated with a range of psychiatric and psychological outcomes, including post-traumatic stress disorder (PTSD), substance abuse, depression, and suicide attempts [2–4]. A variety of risk factors have been identified to be associated with this phenomenon, such as borderline and dependent personality disorders, prior victimisation by IPV, childhood sexual and physical abuse [5], and the use of substances like alcohol, cocaine, and amphetamines [6].

Children raised in violent households—either as direct victims or witnesses—are at heightened risk of internalising violence as a means of asserting power and control in relationships. When such environments coexist with patriarchal cultural systems, the transmission of harmful gender role ideologies across generations is further reinforced [7–9]. These ideologies are shaped by culturally ingrained gender stereotypes that promote the perception of men as dominant providers and women as dependent and subordinate [10,11]. Developmental research suggests that gender-stereotypical thinking emerges early in life and remains remarkably resistant to change, being shaped by family, peers, education, and the media [10,12].

Despite significant progress toward gender equality, traditional gender norms continue to exert detrimental effects across domains such as employment, education, and even legal decision-making [13–16]. Notably, adherence to traditional gender roles has been found to be positively correlated with IPV perpetration [17], and exposure to childhood violence is associated with a greater acceptance of male dominance and a higher likelihood of adult perpetration of IPV [18]. Research further links gender inequality at a social level with elevated IPV rates in both Europe and the United States [19,20].

Additionally, specific offence-supportive beliefs—such as minimising personal responsibility, externalising blame (e.g., on substance use), and holding rigid control-related views—have been associated with IPV [21–23]. While not all individuals exposed to domestic violence become perpetrators [24], such early experiences can indirectly influence future abusive behaviour through the development of legitimising beliefs and attitudes [25].

Endorsement of legitimising beliefs—those that justify, excuse, or trivialise IPV—has been found to vary by gender, age, education, and history of exposure to violence. Men and younger individuals tend to express greater acceptance of IPV, particularly in contexts shaped by patriarchal cultural norms, while higher education appears to act as a protective factor [26–28].

Against this backdrop, the present study aims to examine whether Portuguese IPV offenders endorse legitimising beliefs about IPV, and, if so, to identify which specific beliefs are most prevalent within this population. By shedding light on the attitudinal underpinnings of IPV, this research contributes to a more nuanced understanding of the mechanisms through which cultural, social, and individual factors sustain intimate partner violence.

2. Method

This research was conducted using the existent forensic psychological assessment reports of the Forensic Psychology Office (GPF; Laboratory of Forensic and Psychological Sciences Egas Moniz). Within these existent data, we selected those whereby individuals were assessed using the Belief Scale of Conjugal Violence (E.C.V.C.) [29]. This instrument assesses the presence of intimate partner violence-legitimising beliefs. There are 4 scales that are incorporated into this instrument, the first being legitimising and banalising "minor" violence; the second is legitimising violence due to women's behaviour; the third is legitimising violence because of external factors; and the fourth is legitimising violence to preserve family privacy. Additionally, there is also a total score. Our sample consisted of 45 individuals, including 24 women and 21 men, with ages ranging between 18 and 75 years old (M= 41.40; SD = 13.84). Regarding academic level, this variable included six groups, including primary school (n = 4), middle school (n = 9), junior high school (n = 10), high school (n = 13), bachelor's degree (n = 6), and master's degree (n = 2). The total sample included 16 offenders and 16 non-offenders. As for occupation, this category was divided into specialists in intellectual and scientific activities (n = 3), technicians and intermediate-level professionals (n = 3), administrative personnel (n = 1), personal and protective services workers (n = 6), skilled industrial workers (n = 1), facility and machine operators (n = 3), unskilled workers (n = 9), retired individuals (n = 2), students (n = 3), housekeepers (n = 2), and unemployed individuals (n = 10). Statistical analysis was conducted using IBM SPSS Statistics, Version 29.0 (IBM Corp., Armonk, NY, USA). Due to some of the variables not having a normal distribution, non-parametric tests were used, in particular, Mann–Whitney and Kruskal–Wallis tests.

3. Results and Discussion

The goal of this study is to identify IPV-legitimising beliefs in offenders and which of the four factors is more prevalent within each category.

Table 1 shows significant differences between ECVC factors in different groups, such as academic level, sex, and profession.

Table 1. Results from the statistical analysis.

Variable	Factor 1	Factor 2	Factor 3	Factor 4	Total ECVC Score
Offender vs. non-offenders	U [a] = 134.50 $p = 0.007$	-	-	U [a] = 150.00 $p = 0.031$	U [a] = 149.00 $p = 0.030$
Academic Level	H [b] = 15.20 $p = 0.010$	H [b] = 15.66 $p = 0.008$	F [c] = 5.932 $p < 0.001$	F [c] = 4.635 $p = 0.002$	F [c] = 4.645 $p = 0.002$
Sex	U [a] = 116.50 $p = 0.002$	U [a] = 134.00 $p = 0.011$	-	F [c] = 5.213 $p = 0.028$	F [c] = 6.175 $p = 0.017$
Occupational category	H [b] = 20.673 $p = 0.023$	-	-	-	F [c] = 2.660 $p = 0.018$

[a] Mann–Whitney; [b] Kruskal–Wallis; [c] ANOVA.

The results of our study align with the existing literature, more specifically regarding the main characteristics of offenders with higher IPV-legitimising beliefs. Men present higher levels of IPV-legitimising beliefs, which is corroborated by the literature [10–12]. Research has shown that the influence of the patriarchal characteristics that are still present in society has a significant impact on developing and maintaining these beliefs, more specifically, the provider role that is attributed to men and the expectation of submission by women [11]. Additionally, the previously mentioned beliefs appear to be more prevalent among people with lower educational levels and, therefore, with a professional career in certain professional categories, such as industry workers, machine operators, and those in personal protective services [13–16,28].

4. Conclusions

This study confirms that Portuguese IPV offenders endorse legitimising beliefs, especially those that trivialise "minor" violence and justify it as a way to protect family privacy. These beliefs are more prevalent among men, individuals with lower education levels, and those in manual or protective service jobs—often older or retired individuals. These findings highlight the need for offender programmes to address underlying gender norms, particularly patriarchal beliefs. Prevention strategies should focus on education and gender equality, especially in lower-skilled professions. Ultimately, reducing IPV requires tackling the social and cultural attitudes that support it, through integrated efforts across the justice, education, and public health sectors.

Author Contributions: Conceptualization, M.B.R., I.A., G.S. and R.V.B.; methodology, M.B.R., I.A., G.S. and R.V.B.; formal analysis, M.B.R., I.A., G.S. and R.V.B.; writing—original draft preparation, M.B.R. and I.A.; writing—review and editing, M.B.R. and I.A.; visualisation, R.V.B. and I.A.; supervision, I.A. and R.V.B. All authors have read and agreed to the published version of the manuscript.

Funding: This research received no external funding.

Institutional Review Board Statement: This study is part of a protocol established among the Portuguese Public Prosecutor's Office and Egas Moniz School of Health & Science to assess and analyse the characteristics of offenders in the field of violence. The strictness of ethical and deontological principles is safeguarded as criminal records have restricted access by law (including judicial secrecy). Therefore, all assessed subjects gave their informed consent, and their data were processed anonymously. This study was conducted according to the Declaration of Helsinki and approved by the Egas Moniz Ethics Committee (Process No. 1231/2023), and all ethical standards of scientific research were respected, as was the Code of Ethics of the Order of Portuguese Psychologists and the General Data Protection Regulation.

Informed Consent Statement: Informed consent for participation was obtained from all subjects involved in the study.

Data Availability Statement: The datasets presented in this article are not readily available because some of the information was derived from criminal records.

Conflicts of Interest: The authors declare no conflicts of interest.

References

1. Wenigmann, M.; Weiß, J.; Heidelberg, R. Holding anti-feminist gender role beliefs mediate the relationship between family-related adverse childhood experiences and different forms of intimate partner violence perpetration in adulthood. *J. Crim. Justice* **2024**, *93*, 102214. [CrossRef]
2. Black, M.C.; Basile, K.C.; Breiding, M.J.; Smith, S.G.; Walters, M.L.; Merrick, M.T.; Chen, J.; Stevens, M.R. *The National Intimate Partner and Sexual Violence Survey (NISVS): 2010 Summary Report*; National Center for Injury Prevention and Control, Centers for Disease Control and Prevention: Atlanta, GA, USA, 2011.
3. White, S.J.; Sin, J.; Sweeney, A.; Salisbury, T.; Wahlich, C.; Guevara, C.M.M.; Gillard, S.; Brett, E.; Allwright, L.; Iqbal, N.; et al. Global prevalence and mental health outcomes of intimate partner violence among women: A systematic review and meta-analysis. *Trauma Violence Abus.* **2023**, *25*, 494–511. [CrossRef] [PubMed]
4. World Health Organization. *Global and Regional Estimates of Violence Against Women: Prevalence and Health Effects of Intimate Partner Violence and Non-Partner Sexual Violence*; WHO: Geneva, Switzerland, 2013. Available online: https://apps.who.int/iris/handle/10665/85239 (accessed on 20 June 2025).
5. Okuda, M.; Olfson, M.; Wang, S.; Rubio, J.M.; Xu, Y.; Blanco, C. Correlates of intimate partner violence perpetration: Results from a national epidemiologic survey. *J. Trauma. Stress* **2015**, *28*, 49–56. [CrossRef]
6. Shorey, R.C.; Brasfield, H.; Zapor, H.; Febres, J.; Stuart, G.L. The relation between alcohol use and psychological, physical, and sexual dating violence perpetration among male college students. *Violence Against Women* **2014**, *21*, 151–164. [CrossRef]
7. Chesworth, B.R. Intimate partner violence perpetration: Moving toward a comprehensive conceptual framework. *Partn. Abus.* **2018**, *9*, 75–100. [CrossRef]
8. Dodaj, A. Children witnessing domestic violence. *J. Child. Serv.* **2020**, *15*, 161–174. [CrossRef]
9. Graham-Bermann, S.A.; Brescoll, V. Gender, power, and violence: Assessing the family stereotypes of the children of batterers. *J. Fam. Psychol.* **2000**, *14*, 600–612. [CrossRef]
10. Boehnke, M. Gender role attitudes around the globe: Egalitarian vs. traditional views. *Asian J. Soc. Sci.* **2011**, *39*, 57–74. [CrossRef]
11. Hardesty, J.; Ogolsky, B. A socioecological perspective on intimate partner violence research: A decade in review. *J. Marriage Fam.* **2020**, *82*, 454–477. [CrossRef]
12. Larsen, K.S.; Long, E. Attitudes toward sex-roles: Traditional or egalitarian? *Sex Roles* **1988**, *19*, 1–12. [CrossRef]
13. Castaño, A.M.; Fontanil, Y.; García-Izquierdo, A.L. "Why can't I become a manager?"—A systematic review of gender stereotypes and organizational discrimination. *Int. J. Environ. Res. Public Health* **2019**, *16*, 1813. [CrossRef]
14. Koch, A.J.; D'Mello, S.D.; Sackett, P.R. A meta-analysis of gender stereotypes and bias in experimental simulations of employment decision making. *J. Appl. Psychol.* **2015**, *100*, 128–161. [CrossRef]
15. Schuller, R.A.; McKimmie, B.M.; Masser, B.M.; Klippenstine, M.A. Judgments of sexual assault: The impact of complainant emotional demeanor, gender, and victim stereotypes. *New Crim. Law Rev.* **2010**, *13*, 759–780. [CrossRef]
16. Alan, S.; Ertac, S.; Mumcu, I. Gender stereotypes in the classroom and effects on achievement. *Rev. Econ. Stat.* **2018**, *100*, 876–890. [CrossRef]
17. Spencer, C.M.; Stith, S.M.; Cafferky, B. What puts individuals at risk for physical intimate partner violence perpetration? A meta-analysis examining risk markers for men and women. *Trauma Violence Abus.* **2020**, *23*, 36–51. [CrossRef] [PubMed]
18. Lichter, E.L.; McCloskey, L.A. The effects of childhood exposure to marital violence on adolescent gender-role beliefs and dating violence. *Psychol Women Q.* **2004**, *28*, 344–357. [CrossRef]
19. González, L.; Rodríguez-Planas, N. Gender norms and intimate partner violence. *J. Econ. Behav. Organ.* **2020**, *178*, 223–248. [CrossRef]
20. Willie, T.C.; Kershaw, T.S. An ecological analysis of gender inequality and intimate partner violence in the United States. *Prev. Med.* **2019**, *118*, 257–263. [CrossRef]
21. Babcock, J.C.; Waltz, J.; Jacobson, N.S.; Gottman, J.M. Power and violence: The relation between communication patterns, power discrepancies, and domestic violence. *J. Consult. Clin. Psychol.* **1993**, *61*, 40–50. [CrossRef]
22. Gilchrist, E. The cognition of domestic abusers: Explanations, evidence and treatment. In *Aggressive Offenders' Cognition: Theory, Research and Practice*; Gannon, T.A., Ward, T., Beech, A.R., Fisher, D., Eds.; John Wiley & Sons Ltd.: Chichester, UK, 2007; pp. 247–266. [CrossRef]
23. Prince, J.E.; Arias, I. The role of perceived control and the desirability of control among abusive and nonabusive husbands. *Am. J. Fam. Ther.* **1994**, *22*, 126–134. [CrossRef]
24. Stets, J.E.; Pirog-Good, M.A. Violence in dating relationships. *Soc. Psychol. Q.* **1987**, *50*, 237–246. [CrossRef]

25. Silverman, J.G.; Williamson, G.M. Social ecology and entitlements involved in battering by heterosexual college males: Contributions of family and peers. *Violence Vict.* **1997**, *12*, 147–164. [CrossRef]
26. Han, Y.R.; Jeong, G.H.; Kim, S.J. Factors influencing beliefs about intimate partner violence among adults in South Korea. *Public Health Nurs.* **2017**, *34*, 412–421. [CrossRef]
27. Mota, T. Crenças e Significados da Violência nas Relações de Intimidade em Estudantes Universitários/as. Master's Thesis, Universidade do Porto–Faculdade de Psicologia e de Ciências da Educação, Porto, Portugal, 2021. Available online: https://hdl.handle.net/10216/137702 (accessed on 20 June 2025).
28. Boaventura, B. Motivação Para a Mudança e Crenças Legitimadoras de Violência em Relações de Intimidade. Master's Thesis, Universidade do Minho, Braga, Portugal, 2021.
29. Machado, C.; Matos, M.; Gonçalves, M. *Manual de Escala de Crenças Sobre a Violência Conjugal (E.C.V.C.) e do Inventário de Violência Conjugal (I.V.C.): Escalas de Avaliação e Manual*; Editora Psiquilíbrios: Braga, Portugal, 2008.

medical sciences forum

MDPI

Proceeding Paper

Sexual Harassment in Higher Education Students †

Margarida M. C. Ramos [1,*], Marta Reis [1], Telma C. Almeida [1,2] and Jorge Cardoso [1,2]

[1] Egas Moniz School of Health & Science, Caparica, 2829-511 Almada, Portugal; mreis@egasmoniz.edu.pt (M.R.); talmeida@egasmoniz.edu.pt (T.C.A.); jcardoso@egasmoniz.edu.pt (J.C.)
[2] Egas Moniz Centre for Interdisciplinary Research (CiiEM), Egas Moniz School of Health and Science, Caparica, 2829-511 Almada, Portugal
* Correspondence: margaridamc.ramos@gmail.com
† Presented at the 7th CiiEM International Congress 2025—Empowering One Health to Reduce Social Vulnerabilities, Caparica, Portugal, 2–4 July 2025.

Abstract: Sexual harassment, globally recognized as a complex phenomenon, presents gaps regarding its characteristics and diversity of impacts, particularly in the Portuguese context. This study aims to better understand sexual harassment in Portuguese universities, namely the prevalence of these experiences, their types, perpetrators, and settings, as well as the psychosocial factors associated with them, specifically distress, intrusive negative thoughts, academic engagement, and resilience. Positive correlations were found between unwanted sexual experiences, distress, intrusive negative thoughts, and academic engagement. These findings highlight the need for more effective policies to prevent sexual harassment and for psychological support programs for victims of sexual harassment.

Keywords: sexual harassment; unwanted sexual experiences; higher education students; psychological impact; distress

1. Introduction

In the European Union, from the age of 15, one in every two women has experienced sexual harassment at least once in her lifetime [1]. Sexual harassment can be defined as "any unwanted behaviour of a sexual nature, whether verbal, non-verbal or physical, with the purpose or effect of disturbing or constraining the person, affecting their dignity, or creating an intimidating, hostile, degrading, humiliating or destabilising environment" [2] (p. 1).

Sexual harassment can seriously impact victims in the short and long term, both physically and psychologically, as well as academically [3]. This type of abusive behavior can have significant adverse effects on mental health [4] and is often experienced as a distressing event, which can trigger symptoms of depression, anxiety, stress, rumination, and even post-traumatic stress disorder [3]. When sexual harassment occurs in higher education institutions, it can affect students' overall perception of their academic experience, reducing their commitment, performance, and motivation, contributing to academic disengagement [3]. Resilience has a fundamental role in mitigating the emotional and academic consequences of sexual harassment, with higher levels of resilience being associated with fewer symptoms of distress and rumination [5,6].

This study aims to better understand sexual harassment in the context of higher education in Portugal, namely the prevalence of these experiences, their types, perpetrators, and settings, as well as the psychosocial factors associated with them, namely distress, intrusive negative thoughts, academic engagement, and resilience.

2. Materials and Methods

A sample of 541 students from public and private higher education institutions (M = 22.57, SD = 4.71) participated in the study. The majority were women (n = 420, 77.6%), currently enrolled in bachelor's (n = 271, 50.1%) or master's (n = 175, 32.3%) programs. Participants completed the following self-report instruments: the Sexual Experiences Questionnaire (SEQ) [7,8], the Distress Scale (DS) [9], the Intrusive Negative Thoughts Scale (INTS) [10], the Academic Engagement Questionnaire (AEQ) [3,11], and the Resilience Scale (RS) [12]. The SEQ measures the prevalence of unwanted sexual experiences; the DS evaluates psychological distress; the INTS assesses repetitive and maladaptive negative thoughts; the AEQ measures indicators of academic engagement and disengagement. For this study, the scoring was reversed, meaning that higher scores indicate lower academic engagement; and the RS assesses the individual's ability to cope with adversity through self-determination and adaptability. Descriptive analyses of sociodemographic characteristics and psychological variables were conducted to assess normality and instruments' reliability. All participants gave their consent to participate in this research. The study followed the ethical principles outlined in the Declaration of Helsinki [13] and was approved by the Institutional Review Board of the Egas Moniz School of Health and Science.

3. Results and Discussion

3.1. Prevalence and Characterization of Sexual Harassment Experiences

Considering the sample under study, 56 participants (14.4%) reported having suffered sexual harassment, and the majority were female, with an average age of 21.5 years (SD = 3.30). The majority were studying at public higher education institutions (60.7%), mostly located in the Lisbon Metropolitan Area (75%). A large proportion were currently enrolled in bachelor's (44.6%) or master's (35.7%) programs, particularly in health-related areas (41.1%). Most participants reported being harassed by a male colleague (51.8%), typically during parties on Campus (41.1%) or in classrooms and laboratories (28.6%). In response to these abusive incidents, most pretended not to realize (55.4%), while others expressed immediate discomfort or indignation (41.1%).

Our findings on the prevalence of sexual harassment (14,4%) are consistent with studies carried out in Australia (16.1%) and Norway (24.2%) [14,15]. Most victims were women, reinforcing previous research that highlights the higher exposure of female students to unwanted sexual behaviors [15,16]. This female vulnerability may stem from gender inequalities, traditional gender roles, objectification of women in society, and asymmetrical power relations present in academic institutions [17]. Additionally, the average age of the victims (21.5 years) suggests that younger students are particularly susceptible to these experiences, as supported by other studies [14,15], possibly due to higher vulnerability associated with a transitional stage in the life cycle. Most victims reported being harassed by male colleagues, reflecting gender imbalances in the university context, as reported by earlier studies [16,18]. Sexual harassment occurred mainly at Campus parties, in informal settings with less supervision and alcohol consumption. However, it was also reported in formal settings such as classrooms and laboratories, indicating that sexual harassment is not limited to more casual social contexts [14]. Regarding reactions, most reported pretending not to notice the sexual harassment, revealing a culture of silence, fear of retaliation, and stigma, while others expressed immediate distress or indignation, something that can be understood as a sign of growing empowerment. Similar responses have been documented in previous studies [18].

3.2. Correlation Analyses

The results show that unwanted sexual experiences are positively correlated with distress ($r = 0.26$, $p \leq 0.001$), intrusive negative thoughts ($r = 0.16$, $p = 0.003$), and academic engagement ($r = 0.19$, $p \leq 0.001$). Distress is positively correlated with intrusive negative thoughts ($r = 0.52$, $p \leq 0.001$) and academic engagement ($r = 0.35$, $p \leq 0.001$), and it is negatively correlated with resilience ($r = -0.46$, $p \leq 0.001$). Intrusive negative thoughts are also positively correlated with academic engagement ($r = 0.23$, $p \leq 0.001$) and negatively correlated with resilience ($r = -0.39$, $p \leq 0.001$).

The results of the correlational analyses showed that students who reported more experiences of sexual harassment also reported higher levels of distress and intrusive negative thoughts, which is consistent with previous studies [19,20]. Factors such as the severity of harassment, the aggressor's power, and the presence of threats contribute to increased distress [19]. At the same time, self-blame and rumination about the trauma intensify negative thoughts, anxiety, and depression, exacerbating distress [19,21]. Furthermore, students who reported more experiences of sexual harassment revealed lower academic engagement, consistent with previous studies [22]. Sexual harassment can trigger distress and intrusive negative thoughts that impair students' concentration and focus on academic responsibilities, with a possible negative impact on students' motivation and academic performance [3,22]. Students with higher resilience were found to have lower levels of distress and intrusive negative thoughts. This result, also consistent with the literature [23], suggests that resilience in response to traumatic experiences, such as sexual harassment, can reduce symptoms of depression, anxiety, stress, as well as intrusive negative thoughts. Additionally, resilience can serve as a protective factor, enhancing the ability to cope with such events [24].

3.3. Comparison Analyses

In sexual experiences ($t(386) = -7.37$; $p \leq 0.001$), victims ($M = 33.95$; $SD = 12.45$) had a higher mean score than non-victims ($M = 21.59$; $SD = 3.73$). Similarly, in distress ($t(339) = -3.66$; $p \leq 0.001$), victims ($M = 27.10$; $SD = 7.30$) reported higher levels compared to non-victims ($M = 22.71$; $SD = 7.26$). Regarding academic engagement ($t(386) = -2.61$; $p = 0.009$), victims ($M = 12.98$; $SD = 4.87$) also showed higher mean scores than non-victims ($M = 11.57$; $SD = 3.51$).

Victims of sexual harassment reported higher levels of distress compared to those who had not, which is in line with previous findings [25]. These experiences are perceived as psychologically harmful and can trigger a range of adverse emotional outcomes, such as persistent worry, intrusive thoughts, anxiety, and depression [15,26]. The constant fear of reliving the traumatic experience and a perceived lack of control also contributes to increased levels of distress [27]. Furthermore, the stigma surrounding sexual harassment, including victim-blaming and disbelief, can lead to feelings of isolation and shame, increasing distress [28]. Consistent with findings from previous research [29], the results of our study also showed that victims of sexual harassment reported lower levels of academic engagement compared to those who had not experienced sexual harassment, suggesting that victims may feel less safe in environments where such incidents have occurred. In response, some students may begin avoiding certain campus areas, skip classes, consider changing programs, or even drop out. These factors can reduce academic satisfaction and motivation, ultimately leading to decreased academic engagement.

The study may be limited by a non-representative sample, due to its insufficient size and lack of gender diversity, which restricts the ability to capture the population's diversity.

4. Conclusions

This study highlights the urgent need for effective policies to prevent and respond to sexual harassment. Regular awareness campaigns can help create a safer and more inclusive academic environment. Institutions should also provide psychological support programs specifically for victims of sexual harassment. Promoting resilience may help reduce the impact of distress and intrusive negative thoughts, as well as minimizing academic disengagement. Finally, implementing anonymous and confidential reporting channels is crucial in encouraging victims to come forward.

Author Contributions: Conceptualization, M.M.C.R., M.R., and J.C.; methodology, M.M.C.R., M.R., and J.C.; validation, M.M.C.R., M.R., and J.C.; formal analysis, M.M.C.R., M.R., T.C.A., and J.C.; investigation, M.M.C.R., M.R., and J.C.; data curation, M.M.C.R., M.R., and J.C.; writing—original draft preparation, M.M.C.R., M.R., and J.C.; writing—review and editing, M.M.C.R., M.R., T.C.A., and J.C.; supervision, M.M.C.R., M.R., and J.C.; project administration, M.M.C.R., M.R., and J.C. All authors have read and agreed to the published version of the manuscript.

Funding: This research received no external funding.

Institutional Review Board Statement: The study was conducted in accordance with the Declaration of Helsinki and approved by the Institutional Review Board of Egas Moniz School of Health and Science (protocol code 1307) on [25 January 2024].

Informed Consent Statement: Informed consent for participation was obtained from all subjects involved in the study.

Data Availability Statement: The raw data supporting the conclusions of this article will be made available by the authors on request.

Acknowledgments: The authors would like to express the most profound gratitude to all the participants who voluntarily provided information to this study and consented to their involvement.

Conflicts of Interest: The authors declare no conflicts of interest.

References

1. Latcheva, R. Sexual Harassment in the European Union: A Pervasive but Still Hidden Form of Gender-Based Violence. *J. Interpers. Violence* **2017**, *32*, 1821–1852. [CrossRef]
2. Associação Portuguesa de Apoio à Vítima (APAV). *Assédio no Local de Trabalho*; APAV: Lisboa, Portugal, 2020; Available online: https://apav.pt/apav_v3/images/folhas_informativas/Asse%CC%81dio_no_Trabalho_2020.pdf (accessed on 15 October 2024).
3. Huerta, M.; Cortina, L.M.; Pang, J.S.; Torges, C.M.; Magley, V.J. Sex and Power in the Academy: Modeling Sexual Harassment in the Lives of College Women. *Pers. Soc. Psychol. Bull.* **2006**, *32*, 616–628. [CrossRef]
4. Bucchianeri, M.M.; Eisenberg, M.E.; Wall, M.M.; Piran, N.; Neumark-Sztainer, D. Multiple Types of Harassment: Associations with Emotional Well-Being and Unhealthy Behaviors in Adolescents. *J. Adolesc. Health* **2014**, *54*, 724–729. [CrossRef]
5. Moldovan, O.; Macarie, F. Resilience, Gender Discrimination and Sexual Harassment in Romanian Higher Education. In *Sustainable Development and Resilience of Local Communities and Public Sector Organizations*; Haruța, C., Hințea, C.M., Moldovan, O., Eds.; Accent: Cluj-Napoca, Romania, 2019; pp. 403–422. Available online: https://ssrn.com/abstract=3324639 (accessed on 25 January 2025).
6. Thambo, S.; Tshifhumulo, R.; Amaechi, K.O.; Mabale, D. Resilience in Women—Strategies Female Students Employ to Deal with Online Sexual Harassment. *Afr. J. Gend. Soc. Dev.* **2019**, *8*, 91. [CrossRef]
7. Fitzgerald, L.F.; Shullman, S.L.; Bailey, N.; Richards, M.; Swecker, J.; Gold, Y.; Ormerod, M.; Weitzman, L. The Incidence and Dimensions of Sexual Harassment in Academia and the Workplace. *J. Vocat. Behav.* **1988**, *32*, 152–175. [CrossRef]
8. Fitzgerald, L.F.; Gelfand, M.J.; Drasgow, F. Measuring Sexual Harassment: Theoretical and Psychometric Advances. *Basic Appl. Soc. Psychol.* **1995**, *17*, 425–445. [CrossRef]
9. Kessler, R.; Andrews, G.; Colpe, L.J.; Hiripi, E.; Mroczek, D.K.; Normand, S.L.T.; Walters, E.E.; Zaslavsky, A.M. Short Screening Scales to Monitor Population Prevalences and Trends in Non-Specific Psychological Distress. *Psychol. Med.* **2002**, *32*, 959–976. [CrossRef]

10. Magson, N.R.; Rapee, R.M.; Fardouly, J.; Forbes, M.K.; Richardson, C.E.; Johnco, C.J.; Oar, E.L. Measuring Repetitive Negative Thinking: Development and Validation of the Persistent and Intrusive Negative Thoughts Scale (PINTS). *Psychol. Assess.* **2019**, *31*, 1329. [CrossRef] [PubMed]
11. Cortina, L.M.; Swan, S.; Fitzgerald, L.F.; Waldo, C. Sexual Harassment and Assault: Chilling the Climate for Women in Academia. *Psychol. Women Q.* **1998**, *22*, 419–441. [CrossRef]
12. Wagnild, G.M.; Young, H.M. Development and Psychometric Evaluation of the Resilience Scale. *J. Nurs. Meas.* **1993**, *1*, 165–178. Available online: https://pubmed.ncbi.nlm.nih.gov/7850498/ (accessed on 25 January 2024).
13. World Medical Association. World Medical Association Declaration of Helsinki: Ethical Principles for Medical Research Involving Human Subjects. *JAMA* **2013**, *310*, 2191–2194. [CrossRef]
14. Heywood, W.; Myers, P.; Powell, A.; Meikle, G.; Nguyen, D. *Report on the Prevalence of Sexual Harassment and Sexual Assault among University Students in 2021*; The Social Research Centre: Melbourne, Australia, 2022; Available online: https://universitiesaustralia.edu.au/publication/2021-nsss-national-report/ (accessed on 15 October 2024).
15. Sivertsen, B.; Nielsen, M.B.; Madsen, I.E.; Knapstad, M.; Lønning, K.J.; Hysing, M. Sexual Harassment and Assault among University Students in Norway: A Cross-Sectional Prevalence Study. *BMJ Open* **2019**, *9*, e026993. [CrossRef] [PubMed]
16. Wood, L.; Hoefer, S.; Kammer-Kerwick, M.; Parra-Cardona, J.R.; Busch-Armendariz, N. Sexual Harassment at Institutions of Higher Education: Prevalence, Risk, and Extent. *J. Interpers. Violence* **2021**, *36*, 4520–4544. [CrossRef]
17. Marshall, C.; Dalyot, K.; Galloway, S. Sexual Harassment in Higher Education: Re-Framing the Puzzle of Its Persistence. *J. Policy Pract.* **2014**, *13*, 276–299. [CrossRef]
18. Boskovic, I.; Orthey, R.; Otgaar, H.; Mangiulli, I.; Rassin, E. #StudentsToo. Prevalence of Sexual Assault Reports among Students of Three European Universities and Their Actions Post-Assault. *PLoS ONE* **2023**, *18*, e0283554. [CrossRef]
19. Collinsworth, L.L.; Fitzgerald, L.F.; Drasgow, F. In Harm's Way: Factors Related to Psychological Distress Following Sexual Harassment. *Psychol. Women Q.* **2009**, *33*, 475–490. [CrossRef]
20. Gautam, N.; Sapakota, N.; Shrestha, S.; Regmi, D. Sexual Harassment in Public Transportation among Female Students in Kathmandu Valley. *Risk Manag. Healthc. Policy* **2019**, *12*, 105–113. [CrossRef] [PubMed]
21. Sinclair, L.; Trapnell, P.; Kinsman, L. Making the Personal Political: Personal versus Group-Focused Rumination Following Sexual Harassment. *Sex Roles* **2023**, *89*, 517–538. [CrossRef]
22. Kirkner, A.C.; Lorenz, K.; Mazar, L. Faculty and Staff Reporting & Disclosure of Sexual Harassment in Higher Education. *Gend. Educ.* **2022**, *34*, 199–215. [CrossRef]
23. Jeamjitvibool, T.; Duangchan, C.; Mousa, A.; Mahikul, W. The Association between Resilience and Psychological Distress during the COVID-19 Pandemic: A Systematic Review and Meta-Analysis. *Int. J. Environ. Res. Public Health* **2022**, *19*, 14854. [CrossRef]
24. McBride, H.; Ireland, C. The Impact of Coping Style, Self-Efficacy, Emotional Reaction and Resilience on Trauma Related Intrusive Thoughts. *J. Forensic Pract.* **2016**, *18*, 229–239. [CrossRef]
25. Bastiani, F.; Romito, P.; Saurel-Cubizolles, M.J. Mental Distress and Sexual Harassment in Italian University Students. *Arch. Womens Ment. Health* **2019**, *22*, 229–236. [CrossRef] [PubMed]
26. Fitzgerald, L.F.; Hulin, C.L.; Drasgow, F. The Antecedents and Consequences of Sexual Harassment in Organizations: An Integrated Model. In *Job Stress in a Changing Workforce: Investigating Gender, Diversity, and Family Issues*; Keita, G.P., Hurrell, J.J., Jr., Eds.; American Psychological Association: Washington, DC, USA, 1994; pp. 55–73. [CrossRef]
27. Mushtaq, M.; Sultana, S.; Imtiaz, I. The Trauma of Sexual Harassment and Its Mental Health Consequences among Nurses. *J. Coll. Physicians Surg. Pak.* **2015**, *25*, 675–679. Available online: https://www.researchgate.net/publication/282037857_The_Trauma_of_Sexual_Harassment_and_its_Mental_Health_Consequences_Among_Nurses (accessed on 14 November 2024). [PubMed]
28. De Judicibus, M.; McCabe, M.P. Blaming the Target of Sexual Harassment: Impact of Gender Role, Sexist Attitudes, and Work Role. *Sex Roles* **2001**, *44*, 401–417. [CrossRef]
29. Shad, F.; Khan, A.; Ullah, M.; Nadir, F. Exploring Sexual Harassment and Students' Academic Performance: A Case Study of Business Schools of Peshawar City. *J. Soc. Sci. Rev.* **2023**, *3*, 417–426. [CrossRef]

medical sciences forum

MDPI

Proceeding Paper

A Parkinson's Disease Handwriting Rehabilitation Kit—A Forensic Exploratory Study †

Catarina Santos [1], Vlad Tatarescu [2,3], Mariana Louro [2], Sarah Souza [4], Carina A. Fernandes [5], Carlos Família [2,3,6], Catarina Godinho [3,6], Alexandre Quintas [2,3,6] and Alexandra Bernardo [2,3,6,*]

1 Forensic and Criminal Sciences, Egas Moniz School of Health and Science, Monte de Caparica, 2829-511 Caparica, Portugal; catarinaquiteriosantos@hotmail.com
2 Laboratório de Ciências Forenses e Psicológicas Egas Moniz, Monte de Caparica, 2829-511 Caparica, Portugal; vlad.tatarescu@gmail.com (V.T.); marianalourol@gmail.com (M.L.); carlosfamilia@egasmoniz.edu.pt (C.F.); aquintas@egasmoniz.edu.pt (A.Q.)
3 Instituto Universitário Egas Moniz, Egas Moniz School of Health and Science, Monte de Caparica, 2829-511 Caparica, Portugal; cgodinho@egasmoniz.edu.pt
4 NeuroVida—Clínica de Neurologia, Edifício Atlas III, Miraflores, Av. José Gomes Ferreira 13 Piso 0, NeuroVida, 1495-139 Lisboa, Portugal
5 Instituto NCForenses-Ciências Forenses, R. Pinto Bessa 522 R/C ESQ, 4300-428 Porto, Portugal; cafernandes@ncforenses.pt
6 Egas Moniz Center for Interdisciplinary Research (CiiEM), Monte de Caparica, 2829-511 Caparica, Portugal
* Correspondence: abernardo@egasmoniz.edu.pt
† Presented at the 7th CiiEM International Congress 2025—Empowering One Health to Reduce Social Vulnerabilities, Caparica, Portugal, 2–4 July 2025.

Abstract: Legal documents signed by individuals with Parkinson's disease are often disputed due to inconsistencies in their signatures when compared to those executed prior to the disease. This exploratory study aims to develop a handwriting rehabilitation kit designed to improve fine motor skills in the elderly diagnosed with Parkinson's disease. This study involved ten subjects with a diagnosis of Parkinson's disease, four of whom participated in the rehabilitation program and used the kit, while the remaining six were assigned to the control group. All participants underwent traditional rehabilitation and clinical evaluation before and after the twelve-week intervention, as well as satisfaction questionnaires following the intervention. The main changes observed in the intervention group indicated progress, including a reduction in tremor and bradykinesia. The potential clinical and handwriting benefits, as well as the positive feedback and program adherence from participants, support the development of a user-friendly kit for this subset of the elderly population.

Keywords: neurorehabilitation; occupational therapy; writing training instruments; IADL; graphoscopic assessment keyword

1. Introduction

Graphoscopy is a branch of forensic science that involves the study and analysis of handwriting and provision of scientific forensic reports in legal proceedings [1]. In this context, alterations resulting from neurodegenerative diseases such as Parkinson's disease (PD), which affect motor skills (rigidity, bradykinesia and tremor), can compromise handwriting performance [2]. Evidence suggests that physiotherapy and physical exercise programs can promote the recovery of motor skills, while occupational therapy can facilitate the recovery of handwriting, which in turn can contribute to improvement in instrumental activities of daily living (IADLs) [3,4]. This work aims to develop an at-home self-administered handwriting rehabilitation eco-kit (from disposable clinical materials with recycling potential) designed to improve fine motor skills in the elderly.

2. Materials and Methods

The kit, presented in Figure 1, was created to facilitate at-home self-administration of occupational therapy exercises and improve adherence to the rehabilitation program (RP). The kit consists of 1 ping-pong ball, 1 anti-stress ball, 1 plastic coin, 2 rubber bands, 2 beans and 10 paper clips, along with a registration handbook for handwriting occupational therapy exercises (H2OTEs), which enabled patients to follow the program and perform fine motor exercises (hand manipulation, finger isolation, finger flexion and extension and coordination).

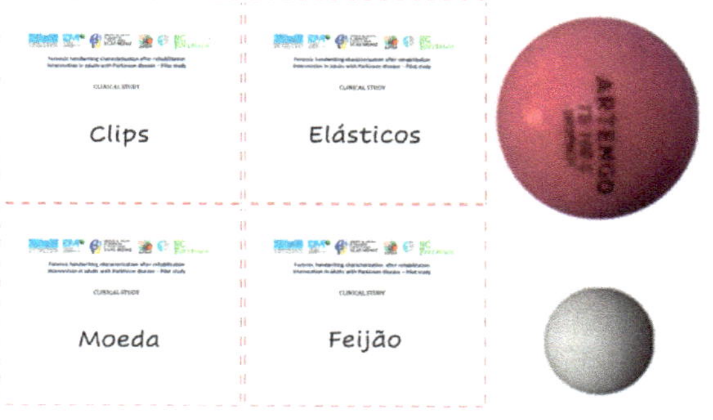

Figure 1. Parkinson's disease handwriting rehabilitation kit.

The procedures implemented in this exploratory study, involving 10 subjects recruited through Clínica de Fisioterapia Egas Moniz at Monte da Caparica, were subject to registration in clinicaltrials.gov (NCT06693401), scientific approval (Egas Moniz Scientific Council) and ethical approval (EM Ethics Committee: protocol code 1171/2023), in accordance with the Declaration of Helsinki (Declaration of 1975, revised in 2000).

The participants were allocated to the control group (CG) or the intervention group (IG) and all of them underwent the traditional physiotherapy rehabilitation program (TPRP) (practice for 1 h, twice a week), which was implemented according to the European Physiotherapy Guideline for Parkinson's Disease [5,6]. The IG also underwent the occupational therapy rehabilitation program (OTRP), which was implemented through workbooks, practiced for 30 min, three times a week [7], and the motor tasks, adapted from Aragon & Kings [8], consisted of performing, 2–3 times a week, exercises included in a workbook (drawing the upper- and lower-case letters of the alphabet guided by dotted lines, writing a sentence with and without spatial limits) and performing 4 groups of fine motor tasks: hand manipulation (2 exercises: (a) hold a dry bean in the palm of the hand, move it to the fingertips and back to the palm of the hand; (b) hold a ping-pong ball in the hand and turn it clockwise and anticlockwise); finger isolation (3 exercises: (a) place the palm and fingers on a table, lift one finger at a time and repeat with all fingers; (b) make an "O" by touching each finger with the thumb; (c) pick up a coin from the table using the thumb and another finger to pinch it, and repeat using each finger); finger flexion and extension (2 exercises: (a) squeeze and release an anti-stress ball; (b) put a rubber band around two fingers at a time and stretch it out); and coordination (1 exercise: make and unmake a chain with 10 clips). All exercises were performed 10 times, in triplicate, for each hand.

The clinical evaluation was performed through the official Portuguese Translation of Movement Disorder Society Unified Parkinson Disease Rating Scale (MDS-UPDRS), which comprises four distinct sections, namely Part I (non-motor aspects of daily life), Part II (motor aspects of daily life), Part III (motor assessment) and Part IV (motor complications) [9]. In this study, the following subgroups were considered: writing (item 2.7); bradykinesia (items 3.4, 3.5 and 3.6) and tremor (items 3.15, 3.16 and 3.17).

To analyze the effect of using the rehabilitation kit in addition to physical therapy on the MDS-UPDRS scores for bradykinesia and tremor, a linear mixed-effects model was developed using the *lmerTest* v.3.1-3 library for R. The model incorporated a fixed effect for time and group and a random intercept for subjects to account for repeated measures. The assumptions of normality and homoscedasticity of the residuals were evaluated through visual inspection of the residual plot, residual quantile–quantile plot and residual histogram, which was performed using the *ggResidPanel* v.0.3.0 library for R. Planned contrasts were subsequently performed to evaluate differences to compare scores between T0 and T1 for each group, and for the slope T0, T1 between groups. These comparisons were performed using the package *emmeans* v.1.8.7 for R, using the Kenward–Roger method to adjust the degrees of freedom and Sidak p-value correction for multiple comparisons.

Adherence to the study was monitored, with records of each assessment at each weekly follow-up visit. The workbooks subjectively assessed performance through a questionnaire after each exercise, in which participants indicated whether they performed the exercises wholly or partially, and all the information was digitally registered.

3. Results

The 10 participants recruited for this study were assigned to the IG and CG while ensuring homogeneity between the two groups, concerning the number of participants, level of education, gender, ethnicity, age, years of PD and other diagnosed pathologies. The main constraint is the limited number of participants, which significantly influences the disparities between initial scores and the values of both intergroup and intragroup interventions. However, despite this constraint, the results presented in Table 1 show that, for the CG MDS-UPDRS scores, there were no significant differences between t0 and t1 for bradykinesia ($t(8) = -0.942$, $p = 0.755$) as well for tremors ($t(8) = 0.000$, $p = 1.000$), while for the IG, there were significant differences between t0 and t1 for bradykinesia ($t(8) = -6.690$, $p < 0.001$) but not for tremors ($t(8) = -1.069$, $p = 0.680$). However, there is an observable decrease in tremors in the IG, which is not observed for the CG. In addition, there was a significant difference between the slope (t0-t1) of both groups for bradykinesia ($t(8) = -4.586$, $p = 0.005$) but not for tremors ($t(8) = -0.828$, $p = 0.816$).

Table 1. MDS-UPDRS scores for bradykinesia and tremor across two assessment moments (t0, t1) and study groups.

	CG		IG	
	t0	t1	t0	t1
Bradykinesia	11.2 (±4.40)	10.3 (±3.67)	11.3 (±4.50)	4.00 (±2.94)
Tremor	2.83 (±3.13)	2.83 (±1.72)	2.25 (±2.63)	1.25 (±1.26)

Concerning adherence and compliance to the study, participants remained engaged for approximately 90.2 days throughout the study and most exercises were completed to a high degree, particularly in categories such as "Hand manipulation," "Finger isolation," "Finger flexion and extension," and "Coordination", as shown in Table 2.

Table 2. Completeness of exercise performance in IG.

Exercise	Completely	Partially	Not Done
Hand manipulation	67.1%	21.1%	11.8%
Finger isolation	86.7%	13.1%	0.2%
Finger flexion and extension	72.5%	26.8%	0.7%
Coordination	97.9%	0.0%	2.1%
Handwriting	96.4%	3.3%	0.2%

4. Conclusions

These preliminary results indicate that individuals with Parkinson's disease who participate in a handwriting rehabilitation program can improve their graphomotor skills, which may aid in recovering their handwriting abilities. Moreover, performing the exercises included in the developed kit results in a significant decrease in bradykinesia and a visible decrease in tremors compared to physiotherapy alone. However, future studies should include a larger sample size to confirm these findings and to better understand the variability in handwriting among people with Parkinson's disease. In addition, based on the potentially beneficial clinical results and the qualitative feedback from the participants' satisfaction questionnaires, which revealed a high level of adherence and satisfaction, it is intended to improve the current kit using a sustainable approach by utilizing disposable hospital waste, converting it into an eco-friendly kit before its future clinical implementation. According to the clinic staff, the most commonly discarded items are disposable bibs, face masks, rubber gloves and surgical sleeves, which, after decontamination and recycling programs, will be explored for conversion into 3D printing filament and production of several kit components.

Author Contributions: Conceptualization, A.B., C.A.F., C.F., C.G., A.Q.; methodology, A.B., C.A.F., C.F., C.G.; software, V.T.; validation, M.L., V.T., C.S.; formal analysis, M.L., V.T., C.S.; investigation, V.T.; resources, C.G.; writing—original draft preparation, M.L.; writing—review and editing, S.S., C.A.F., C.F., C.G., C.A.F., A.Q., A.B.; supervision, A.B., C.A.F., C.F., C.G.; project administration, A.B., C.G. All authors have read and agreed to the published version of the manuscript.

Funding: This research received no external funding.

Institutional Review Board Statement: The study was conducted in accordance with the Declaration of Helsinki and approved by the Ethics Committee of Egas Moniz (protocol code 1171/2023 and date of approval 01/2023) for studies involving humans.

Informed Consent Statement: Informed consent for participation was obtained from all subjects involved in the study.

Data Availability Statement: The raw data supporting the conclusions of this article will be made available by the authors on request.

Acknowledgments: We would like to acknowledge the Laboratório de Ciências Forenses e Psicológicas Egas Moniz (LCFPEM), Clínica de Fisioterapia Egas Moniz and Egas Moniz School of Health and Science.

Conflicts of Interest: The authors declare no conflicts of interest.

References

1. Bensefia, A.; Paquet, T.; Heutte, L. Handwriting analysis for writer verification. In Proceedings of the Ninth International Workshop on Frontiers in Handwriting Recognition, Kokubunji, Japan, 26–29 October 2004; pp. 196–201. [CrossRef]
2. Impedovo, D.; Pirlo, G. Dynamic Handwriting analysis for the assessment of neurodegenerative diseases: A pattern recognition perspective. *IEEE Rev. Biomed. Eng.* **2018**, *12*, 209–220. [CrossRef] [PubMed]

3. Rosário, A.F.L. The Efficacy of Exercise Interventions for People with Parkinson's Disease: A Systematic Review and Meta-Analysis Ana Filipa Rosário. 2018. Available online: http://hdl.handle.net/10451/39136 (accessed on 18 May 2025).
4. Foster, E.R.; Carson, L.G.; Archer, J.; Hunter, E.G. Occupational Therapy Interventions for Instrumental Activities of Daily Living for Adults with Parkinson's Disease: A Systematic Review. *Am. J. Occup. Ther.* **2021**, *75*, 7503190030. [CrossRef] [PubMed]
5. Keus, S.; Munneke, M.; Graziano, M.; Paltamaa, J.; Pelosin, E.; Domingos, J.; Brühlmann, S.; Ramaswamy, B.; Prins, J.; Struiksma, C.; et al. European Physiotherapy Guideline for Parkinson's Disease Developed with Twenty European Professional Associations. 2014. Available online: www.parkinsonnet.info/euguideline (accessed on 18 May 2025).
6. Osborne, J.A.; Botkin, R.; Colon-Semenza, C.; DeAngelis, T.R.; Gallardo, O.G.; Kosakowski, H.; Martello, J.; Pradhan, S.; Rafferty, M.; Readinger, J.L.; et al. Physical Therapist Management of Parkinson Disease: A Clinical Practice Guideline from the American Physical Therapy Association. *Phys. Ther.* **2021**, *102*, pzab302. [CrossRef] [PubMed]
7. Rochester, L.; Nieuwboer, A.; Lord, S. Physiotherapy for Parkinson's disease: Defining evidence within a framework for intervention. *Neurodegener. Dis. Manag.* **2011**, *1*, 57–65. [CrossRef]
8. Aragon, A.; Kings, J. *Occupational Therapy for People with Parkinson's*, 2nd ed.; Royal College of Occupational Therapists: London, UK, 2018.
9. Soares, T.; Vale, T.C.; Guedes, L.C.; Maciel, R.O.; Antunes, A.P.; Camargos, S.; Valadas, A.; Coelho, M.; Godinho, C.; Maia, D.; et al. MDS-UPDRS Portuguese Validation Study Group. Validation of the Portuguese MDS-UPDRS: Challenges to Obtain a Scale Applicable to Different Linguistic Cultures. *Mov. Disord. Clin. Pract.* **2025**, *12*, 34–42. [CrossRef] [PubMed]

medical sciences forum

MDPI

Proceeding Paper

Graphoscopic Evaluation After a Fine Motor Skill Rehabilitation Program in Parkinson's Disease—Exploratory Study †

Mariana Louro [1], Vlad Tatarescu [1,2], Catarina Santos [3], Sarah Souza [4], Carina A. Fernandes [5], Carlos Família [1,2,6], Catarina Godinho [2,6], Alexandre Quintas [1,2,6] and Alexandra Bernardo [1,2,6,]*

1 Laboratório de Ciências Forenses e Psicológicas Egas Moniz, Monte de Caparica, 2829-511 Caparica, Portugal; marianalouro1@gmail.com (M.L.); vlad.tatarescu@gmail.com (V.T.); carlosfamilia@egasmoniz.edu.pt (C.F.); aquintas@egasmoniz.edu.pt (A.Q.)
2 Egas Moniz School of Health and Science, Instituto Universitário Egas Moniz, Monte de Caparica, 2829-511 Caparica, Portugal; cgodinho@egasmoniz.edu.pt
3 Forensic and Criminal Sciences BsC, Egas Moniz School of Health and Science, Monte de Caparica, Caparica, 2829-511 Almada, Portugal; catarinaquiteriosantos@hotmail.com
4 NeuroVida—Clínica de Neurologia, Edifício Atlas III, Miraflores, Av. José Gomes Ferreira 13 Piso 0, NeuroVida, 1495-139 Lisboa, Portugal; sarahsouza@neurovida.pt
5 Instituto NCForenses—Ciências Forenses, R. Pinto Bessa 522 R/C ESQ, 4300-428 Porto, Portugal; cafernandes@ncforenses.pt
6 Egas Moniz Center for Interdisciplinary Research (CiiEM), Egas Moniz School of Health & Science, Caparica, 2829-511 Almada, Portugal
* Correspondence: abernardo@egasmoniz.edu.pt
† Presented at the 7th CiiEM International Congress 2025—Empowering One Health to Reduce Social Vulnerabilities, Caparica, Portugal, 2–4 July 2025.

Abstract: Individuals with Parkinson's disease often face legal disputes over documents signed before the ongoing disease, since fine motor skill changes can lead to alterations in handwriting. Generally, rehabilitation programs focus on mobility in the lower limbs; however, these individuals also face challenges involving the control of fine motor skills, such as handwriting and maintaining their graphic identity. The aim of this exploratory study is to evaluate the effect of a fine motor skill rehabilitation program on the handwriting of these individuals. This study involved 10 subjects with a diagnosis of Parkinson's disease, four of whom participated in the rehabilitation program, while the remaining six were allocated to the control group. All participants were instructed to write specific sentences before and after the twelve-week intervention. The main qualitative changes observed between groups after the graphoscopic analysis were in features such as tremors, retouching/overwriting, size, legibility, and line quality.

Keywords: neurorehabilitation; occupational therapy; fine motor skills; graphoscopic analysis; signature changes

1. Introduction

Handwriting identification and the determination of authenticity of signatures are complex subjects. However, they become more challenging when the documents are signed by individuals with a neurological condition, such as Parkinson's disease, since it can lead to inconsistencies in their signature when compared to those executed prior to the disease [1,2]. This disorder can lead to progressive alterations in handwriting due to bradykinesia, tremor, and rigidity, which limit movement, contribute to muscular pain, and compromise the control of fine motor skills [3]. Since handwriting is a skill that requires muscular movements and coordination, these outcomes have an impact on daily challenges. For instance, potential legal implications involving the control of fine motor skills, such as handwriting, and preserving the graphic identity of these individuals [1]. In recent years, there has been growing evidence suggesting that nonpharmacological interventions including different rehabilitative approaches can improve functional activities in individuals with Parkinson's Disease [4]. However, these studies mainly focus on gait and balance, despite handwriting deficits being very common in Parkison's Disease. The studies assessing handwriting in individuals with Parkinson's Disease usually use kinematic analysis or explore modulating factors such as cues, feedback, or dual tasks [5], but only a few studies investigated the effects of a training on handwriting or used specific outcome measures of handwriting in rehabilitation studies [6]. Thus, the aim of this study is to evaluate the effect of a fine motor skill rehabilitation program on the handwriting of individuals with Parkinson's disease.

2. Materials and Methods

This exploratory study employs a design, as illustrated in Figure 1, involving 10 subjects with a diagnosis of Parkinson's disease, recruited through Clínica de Fisioterapia Egas Moniz at Monte da Caparica. All participants were fully briefed on the conditions under which they would perform the tests and the rehabilitation program procedures and signed informed consent forms. The collection, processing, and dissemination of data were carried out anonymously. The procedures implemented in this exploratory study were subject to registration in clinicaltrials.gov (NCT06693401), scientific approval by the Egas Moniz Scientific Council, and ethical approval by the EM Ethics Committee (protocol code 1171/2023), in accordance with the Declaration of Helsinki (Declaration of 1975, revised in 2000).

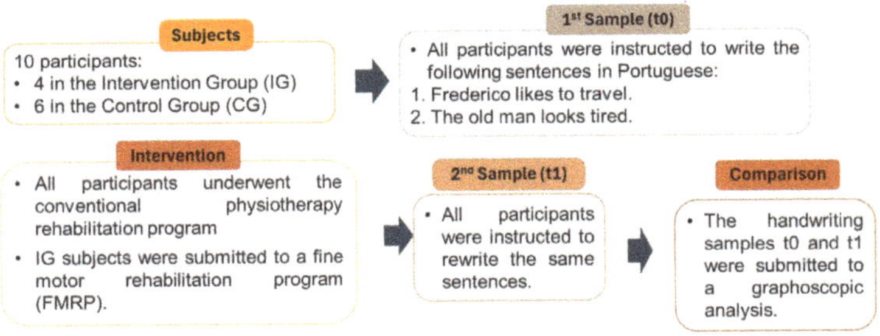

Figure 1. Pilot study design.

The participants were allocated to the Control Group (CG) or the Intervention Group (IG) according to their convenience. A traditional physiotherapy rehabilitation program (TPRP) (practice for 1h, twice a week) was implemented according to the European Physiotherapy Guideline for Parkinson's Disease [7,8]. The Occupational therapy rehabilitation program (OTRP) was implemented through workbooks, practice for 30 min, three times a week [9] and the motor tasks, adapted from Aragon & Kings [10], and consists of performing, 2–3 times a week, exercises included in a workbook (drawing the upper and lower case letters of the alphabet guided by dotted lines, writing a sentence with and without spatial limits), and performing 4 groups of fine motor tasks: hand manipulation (2 exercises: (a) hold a dry bean in the palm of the hand, move it to the fingertips and back to the palm of the hand, (b) hold a ping-pong ball in the hand and turn it clockwise and anticlockwise); finger isolation (3 exercises: (a) place the palm and fingers on a table, lift one finger at a time and repeat with all fingers, (b) make an "O" by touching each finger with the thumb, (c) pick up a coin from the table using the thumb and another finger to pinch it, and repeat using each finger); finger flexion and extension (2 exercises: (a) squeeze and release an anti-stress ball, (b) put a rubber band around two fingers at a time and stretch it out); and coordination (1 exercise: do and undo a chain with 10 clips). All exercises were performed 10 times, in triplicate, for each hand.

The forensic handwriting analysis involved a comparison between t0 and t1 within each group in order to identify potential changes that occurred in the subjects' handwriting over the twelve-week period. Subsequently, an inter-group comparison of the results was carried out to assess the differences in handwriting between the groups, Figure 1.

3. Results

The comparison between the Intervention Group (IG) and the Control Group (CG) revealed that the main qualitative changes observed were in features such as tremors, with a tendency to decrease in the IG and to increase in the CG; retouching/overwriting, where a tendency to decrease was observed in the IG and no changes were observed in CG; size, where no tendency was observed in IG, while an increase was observed in CG; and in line quality, where a better legibility and execution of the letters was achieved in the IG, while the legibility and letters execution worsened in CG. The results of all the comparisons carried out are presented in Table 1.

Table 1. Results of the comparisons of IG and CG handwriting features after the fine motor rehabilitation program.

Features	Intervention Group—IG	Control Group—CG
Tremor	Decreased	Increased
Retouching/ Overwriting	General decrease	Inconsistent (no changes, decrease, and increase)
Size	Inconsistent (decrease and increase)	Increase
Pen Lifts	Mostly no changes	Mostly no changes
Calligraphic box	Sinuous	Sinuous
Baseline	Inconsistent (horizontal, descending, and ascending)	Inconsistent (horizontal and descending)
Slant	Mostly mixed	Mostly mixed
Legibility	Better Legibility	Worse Legibility
Line Quality	Better line quality in letter execution	Worse line quality in letter execution

The reduced sample size and convenience-based recruitment constitute a clear limitation which does not allow the study results' extrapolation, although they validate the methodology and experimental design. While these findings offer valuable preliminary insights, future work should include a larger and heterogeneous sample to ensure greater validity and applicability of the research's results.

4. Conclusions

These preliminary results suggest that individuals with Parkinson's disease engaging in a handwriting rehabilitation program can improve their graphomotor skills, which will promote the recovery of handwriting performance and graphic identity.

In future work, a larger sample size would be desirable to validate these results and to enhance the characterization of variability in Parkinson's disease handwriting.

Author Contributions: Conceptualization, A.B., C.A.F., C.F., C.G. and A.Q.; methodology, A.B., C.A.F., C.F. and C.G.; software, V.T.; validation, M.L., V.T. and C.S.; formal analysis, M.L., V.T. and C.S.; investigation, V.T.; resources, C.G.; writing—original draft preparation, M.L.; writing—review and editing, S.S., C.A.F., C.F., C.G., C.A.F., A.Q. and A.B.; supervision, A.B., C.A.F., C.F. and C.G.;

project administration, A.B. and C.G. All authors have read and agreed to the published version of the manuscript.

Funding: This research received no external funding.

Institutional Review Board Statement: The study was conducted in accordance with the Declaration of Helsinki, and approved by the Ethics Committee of Egas Moniz (protocol code 1171/2023 and date of approval 01/2023).

Informed Consent Statement: Informed consent for participation was obtained from all subjects involved in the study.

Data Availability Statement: The raw data supporting the conclusions of this article will be made available by the authors on request.

Acknowledgments: Laboratório de Ciências Forenses e Psicológicas Egas Moniz (LCFPEM), Clínica de Fisioterapia Egas Moniz and Egas Moniz School of Health and Science.

Conflicts of Interest: The authors declare no conflicts of interest.

References

1. Hilton, O. Influence of age and illness on handwriting: Identification problems. *Forensic Sci.* **1977**, *9*, 161–172. [CrossRef]
2. Hilton, O. Some Basic Rules for the Identification of Handwriting. *J. Am. Soc. Questioned Doc. Exam.* **2001**, *4*, 95–100. [CrossRef]
3. Caligiuri, M.P.; Mohammed, L.A. Neurological Disease and Motor Control. In *The Neuroscience of Handwriting: Applications for Forensic Document Examination*; Caligiuri, M.P., Mohammed, L.A., Eds.; CRC Press: Boca Raton, FL, USA, 2012; pp. 57–69.
4. Abbruzzese, G.; Marchese, R.; Avanzino, L.; Pelosin, E. Rehabilitation for Parkinson's disease: Current outlook and future challenges. *Park. Relat. Disord.* **2016**, *22*, S60–S64. [CrossRef] [PubMed]
5. Cassimatis, C.; Liu, K.P.; Fahey, P.; Bissett, M. The effectiveness of external sensory cues in improving functional performance in individuals with Parkinson's disease: A systematic review with meta-analysis. *Int. J. Rehabil. Res.* **2016**, *39*, 211–218. [CrossRef] [PubMed]
6. Collett, J.; Franssen, M.; Winward, C.; Izadi, H.; Meaney, A.; Mahmoud, W.; Bogdanovic, M.; Tims, M.; Wade, D.; Dawes, H. A long-term self-managed handwriting intervention for people with Parkinson's disease: Results from the control group of a phase II randomized controlled trial. *Clin. Rehabil.* **2017**, *31*, 1636–1645. [CrossRef] [PubMed]
7. Keus, S.; Munneke, M.; Graziano, M.; Paltamaa, J.; Pelosin, E.; Domingos, J.; Brühlmann, S.; Ramaswamy, B.; Prins, J.; Struiksma, C.; et al. European Physiotherapy Guideline for Parkinson's Disease Developed with Twenty European Professional Associations. 2014. Available online: www.parkinsonnet.info/euguideline (accessed on 17 May 2025).
8. Osborne, J.A.; Botkin, R.; Colon-Semenza, C.; Deangelis, T.R.; Gallardo, O.G.; Kosakowski, H.; Martello, J.; Pradhan, S.; Rafferty, M.; Readinger, J.L.; et al. Physical Therapist Management of Parkinson Disease: A Clinical Practice Guideline from the American Physical Therapy Association. In *Physical Therapy*; Oxford University Press: Oxford, UK, 2022; Volume 102. [CrossRef]
9. Rochester, L.; Nieuwboer, A.; Lord, S. Physiotherapy for Parkinson's disease: Defining evidence within a framework for intervention. *Neurodegener. Dis. Manag.* **2011**, *1*, 57–65. [CrossRef]
10. Aragon, A.; Kings, J. *Occupational Therapy for People with Parkinson's*, 2nd ed.; Royal College of Occupational Therapists: London, UK, 2018.

medical sciences forum

MDPI

Proceeding Paper

The Impact of a Modular Curriculum on Veterinary Students' Quality of Life and Academic Knowledge: Proof of Concept †

Bárbara Gonçalves *,‡, Joana Moreira da Silva ‡, Maria Soares, Rita Pequito, Lara Alves, Liliana Silva, Alexandre Trindade and Manuel Pequito *

Egas Moniz Center for Interdisciplinary Research (CiiEM), Egas Moniz School of Health and Science, 2829-511 Caparica, Portugal; jcsilva@egasmoniz.edu.pt (J.M.d.S.); msoares@egasmoniz.edu.pt (M.S.); mrpequito@egasmoniz.edu.pt (R.P.); lalves@egasmoniz.edu.pt (L.A.); lmsilva@egasmoniz.edu.pt (L.S.); atrindade@egasmoniz.edu.pt (A.T.)

* Correspondence: bgoncalves@egasmoniz.edu.pt (B.G.); mpequito@egasmoniz.edu.pt (M.P.)

† Presented at the 7th CiiEM International Congress 2025—Empowering One Health to Reduce Social Vulnerabilities, Caparica, Portugal, 2–4 July 2025.

‡ These authors contributed equally to this work.

Abstract: This study examined quality of life and deep learning among 109 veterinary medicine students across three cohorts (2021–2023) in an integrated modular curriculum in Portugal. Quality of life was measured three times per academic year using the WHOQOL-BREF, whereas deep learning was assessed twice yearly via assessment tests. The results revealed consistently low scores in the psychological domain of the quality-of-life assessment and a noticeable decline in both quality of life and assessment tests during the second year. These findings highlight the need to monitor student well-being and adapt teaching strategies to sustain motivation and academic success.

Keywords: well-being; veterinary students; assessment test; modular curriculum

1. Introduction

The educational landscape has shifted from traditional lectures to active learning, fostering greater student engagement and academic success [1]. This transition attempts to reduce surface learning to promote deep learning, which focuses on understanding, critical thinking, and problem solving rather than mere memorisation [1]. Student motivation drives deep learning, which is impacted by both individual and institutional elements such as the learning environment and teaching strategies, including learning climate, course content, and curriculum design [2].

One innovative approach for curriculum design is a modular curriculum, where students study one subject at a time during the semester. It offers different formats such as sequential, integrative, or integrated approaches that combine theory with practice [3]. Understanding how various factors, such as students' psychological well-being, impact academic performance is essential. Specifically, the well-being of veterinary medicine students is an increasing concern, with rising reports of high stress levels, poor well-being, and depression [4–6]. These outcomes are mostly attributed to the intense academic pressure and high expectations [6].

The Egas Moniz School of Health and Science launched its veterinary medicine programme in the 2021–2022 academic year and has designed it to achieve Day One Competencies after the six-year course. The veterinary course is set on an integrated modular programme, with a strong practical component. It is the first Portuguese institution to adopt this innovative curriculum in veterinary education, striking a balance between contact hours and students' well-being. The latter is critical for maintaining motivation and learning quality. The purpose of this study was to understand how students navigate the course and manage academic demands alongside their personal well-being, as well as to assess their level of deep learning, with the aim of enhancing teaching practices and fostering a supportive learning environment.

2. Materials and Methods

Sample: A total of 109 veterinary medicine students enrolled between the 2021–2022 and 2023–2024 academic years participated in this study. The students were divided into cohorts, according to their entrance year for the course: 2021 cohort, 2022 cohort, and 2023 cohort.

Quality-of-life assessment: Student quality of life was assessed using the WHOQOL-BREF questionnaire at three time points in each academic year: September (start of school), January (end of 1st semester), and June (end of 2nd semester). The questionnaire has 26 items and evaluates four domains: physical, psychological, social relationships, and environmental. Each item was rated on a 5-point Likert scale. Domain scores were calculated according to the *WHOQOL* manual [7].

Study design for post-curricular evaluation: A twice-yearly evaluation was conducted at the beginning of each semester to evaluate the completed curricular units (CUs) per semester, to assess students' deep learning. The test comprised multiple-choice, true/false, and open-response questions; was developed in collaboration with several lecturers from the Egas Moniz School of Health & Science involved in different CUs; and was conducted via an online platform.

Descriptive statistics: Means and standard deviations (SD) were calculated for post-test and quality-of-life questionnaires.

3. Results and Discussion

This study analysed well-being scores and academic assessments of veterinary medicine students across three cohorts. As data collection began in June, only this time point was available for the 2021–2022 cohort, with earlier data missing. Additionally, as the study is ongoing, June data are not yet available for the 4th, 3rd, and 2nd years of the 2021, 2022, and 2023 cohorts, respectively, and are therefore not included.

3.1. Well-Being

As shown in Table 1, among the 109 students enrolled, adherence rates to the WHOQOL-BREF were above 86% at all points, except for the 2021 cohort in the 2nd year (September), which had an adherence rate of 67%.

Table 1. Well-being scores. Means and SD of WHOQOL-BREF scores for veterinary medicine students in the 2021, 2022, and 2023 cohorts. T indicates the total number of students enrolled and *n* the number of students who completed the questionnaire.

Domain/Cohort		**2021 (T = 30)**		**2022 (T = 49)**		**2023 (T = 30)**
	1st year	2nd year (*n* = 20)	3rd year (*n* = 26)	1st year (*n* = 46)	2nd year (*n* = 48)	1st year (*n* = 27)
			September			
Physical	-	68.67 ± 11.96	71.97 ± 13.98	75.23 ± 11.07	68.11 ± 14.48	71.43 ± 11.38
Psychological	-	62.71 ± 14.46	69.07 ± 13.70	68.29 ± 13.48	63.81 ± 15.81	66.82 ± 14.03
Social Relations	-	72.92 ± 16.86	73.07 ± 16.67	76.27 ± 12.66	72.22 ± 13.35	68.21 ± 20.29
Environmental	-	72.81 ± 10.09	75.6 ± 14.89	76.63 ± 9.36	72.85 ± 12.38	71.88 ± 10.07

Table 1. *Cont.*

Domain/Cohort		2021 (T = 30)		2022 (T = 49)		2023 (T = 30)
Domain/Cohort	January					
	1st year	2nd year (*n* = 30)	3rd year (*n* = 26)	1st year (*n* = 50)	2nd year (*n* = 43)	1st year (*n* = 33)
Physical	-	70.35 ± 12.56	68.81 ± 15.47	73.64 ± 13.14	68.85 ± 14.96	70.24 ± 14.73
Psychological	-	66.38 ± 12.38	66.02 ± 13.93	68.1 ± 13.59	63.76 ± 18.71	63.13 ± 15.17
Social Relations	-	73.33 ± 17.42	75.00 ± 22.83	77.17 ± 12.69	71.12 ± 16.19	70.20 ± 20.23
Environmental	-	74.27 ± 12.02	74.4 ± 12.41	74.19 ± 11.94	73.77 ± 13.54	69.32 ± 11.32
Domain/Cohort	June					
	1st year (*n* = 28)	2nd year (*n* = 26)	3rd year (*n* = 24)	1st year (*n* = 47)	2nd year (*n* = 50)	1st year (*n* = 25)
Physical	72.06 ± 13.43	71.43 ± 13.32	85.42 ± 14.89	69.45 ± 15.11	64.93 ± 17.54	72.43 ± 15.52
Psychological	68.15 ± 14.66	70.03 ± 14.09	68.93 ± 15.39	65.78 ± 15.99	61.67 ± 18.71	66.33 ± 16.13
Social Relations	77.97 ± 18.03	75 ± 13.54	77.08 ± 16.35	73.40 ± 17.08	71.67 ± 17.58	71.33 ± 21.79
Environmental	71.76 ± 13.78	73.52 ± 12.19	79.9 ± 12.83	75.46 ± 11.56	70.19 ± 15.48	72.25 ± 15.86

In Table 1, in September, at the beginning of the first semester, the lowest scores across all cohorts and years were observed in the psychological domain (PD), ranging from 62.71 to 69.07. In contrast, the highest scores were found in the environmental domain, ranging from 71.88 to 76.63. For the 2021 cohort, a slight increase in all domains was observed in both the second and third years. Conversely, the 2022 cohort showed a decline across all domains in both the first and second years.

In January, the lowest scores were again observed in the PD, ranging from 63.13 to 68.1. For the 2021 cohort, a slight decrease was noted in the physical domain during the second and third years. In contrast, the 2022 cohort continued to exhibit a decline across all domains in both the first and second years.

In June, a similar behaviour was observed, as the lowest scores were again observed in the PD, ranging from 61.67 to 70.03. For the 2021 cohort, a slight decrease followed by an increase was observed across the first, second, and third years in the physical and social relations domains. Similar behaviour to the previous time points was observed for the 2022 cohort.

Overall, the PD domain has the lowest score across the three time points. This domain measures negative feelings, cognitive functions such as concentration, and body appearance. The WHOQOL questionnaire has previously been used to assess the well-being of veterinary students. The scores in our study were higher than those reported in these studies, as the highest score they reported was 63.57 [4,8]. Furthermore, better academic performance was associated with greater quality of life in most domains [4].

3.2. Assessment Test

A surprise assessment test was administered each semester for the veterinary medicine students across the three cohorts. The adherence rate to the assessment test was always above 83%, except in the first semester of the third year of the 2021 cohort, which the adherence rate was 56%. The test was scored on a scale of 0–20, and the mean score for each CU and semester was calculated. These results are presented in Figure 1.

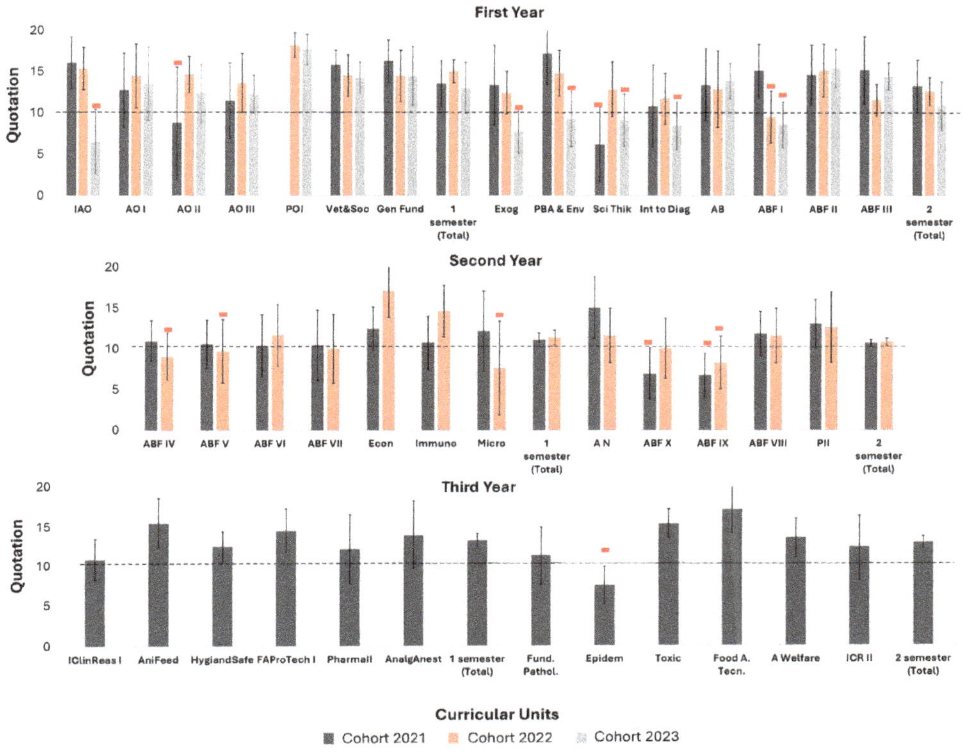

Figure 1. Means and SD of various curricular units in the 1st, 2nd, and 3rd years of the 2021 cohort, the 1st and 2nd years of the 2022 cohort, and the 1st year of the 2023 cohort. The mean scores of the CUs per semester are also presented. The red symbol '-' indicates a negative mean value. A dashed line at value of 10 was introduced to visualise the negative CUs.

As shown in Figure 1, the assessment results revealed that some CUs consistently had negative mean scores. Notably, certain CUs present low scores across multiple cohorts. For example, Scientific Thinking (Sci Think) and Animal Body Function I (ABF I) had low average scores in the 1st year for both the 2022 and 2023 cohorts, while Animal Body Function IX (ABF IX) exhibits similar patterns in the 2nd year for the 2021 and 2022 cohorts. When comparing mean scores across semesters, a decline is evident in the second year. For the 2021 cohort, the average decreased from 13.52 (SD = 2.8) in the first semester to 11.09 (SD = 0.8), and from 13.25 (SD = 3.2) to 10.70 (SD = 3.3) in the second semester. A similar trend was observed in the 2022 cohort: from 15.06 (SD = 1.4) to 11.41 (SD = 3.1) in the first semester, and from 12.64 (SD = 1.7) to 10.84 (SD = 1.5) in the second semester. As the study progresses, we intend to have enough data to try and correlate the grades scored on the assessment tests with the well-being results, thus showcasing how the well-being of students can have an impact on their academic performance.

4. Conclusions

The quality of life varies across cohorts; however, it appears to decrease during the second year. This decline was similar regardless of the time point. Additionally, a decrease in the assessment results was also found in the second year; however, a correlation between these two scores is not yet possible, as the study is ongoing.

Since high stress and poor well-being have been reported among veterinary medicine students, it is important to continue measuring these conditions throughout the veterinary programme. If necessary, Egas Moniz should implement strategies to improve the learning environment and provide support to students to prevent and/or reduce stress. The results obtained in this pilot study support the need to continue with the study to improve the learning environment.

Author Contributions: Conceptualization, M.P., A.T. and R.P.; methodology, M.P., A.T., R.P., L.A. and L.S.; formal analysis, B.G., J.M.d.S. and M.S.; investigation, B.G., J.M.d.S., M.S., M.P., A.T., L.S., L.A. and R.P.; writing—original draft preparation, B.G. and J.M.d.S.; writing—review and editing, M.S., M.P., A.T., L.S., L.A. and R.P.; supervision, M.P. and A.T.; project administration, M.P. and A.T. All authors have read and agreed to the published version of the manuscript.

Funding: This research received no external funding.

Institutional Review Board Statement: The study was conducted in accordance with the Declaration of Helsinki and approved by the Ethics Committee of Egas Moniz School of Health & Science protocol code 1597 and April 2025. The data were collected from 2021 to 2023 in an academic environment. This is a retrospective study, with the data fully anonymised prior to analysis. No personal identifiers were used, and the study complied with all applicable ethical standards for the secondary use of previously collected educational and/or health-related data.

Informed Consent Statement: Verbal informed consent was obtained rather than written because the data were collected from an academic environment, all data were fully anonymous, no personal or identifiable information was collected, and the study involved minimal risk to participants.

Data Availability Statement: Data are unavailable due to ethical restrictions; furthermore, this is an ongoing study.

Acknowledgments: We want to acknowledge Paulo Fernandes and Bárbara Fernandes for the technical support.

Conflicts of Interest: The authors declare no conflicts of interest.

References

1. Fornari, A.; Poznanski, A. *How-to Guide for Active Learning*; International Association of Medical Science: Huntington, WV, USA, 2015; ISBN 978-1-495-17341-7.
2. McCormick, A.C.; Kinzie, J.; Gonyea, R.M. Student engagement: Bridging research and practice to improve the quality of undergraduate education. In *Higher Education: Handbook of Theory and Research*; Paulsen, M.B., Ed.; Springer: Dordrecht, The Netherlands, 2013; Volume 28, pp. 47–92. [CrossRef]
3. Brecher, B. Complicity and modularisation: How universities were made safe for the market. *Crit. Q.* **2005**, *47*, 72–82. [CrossRef]
4. Chattu, V.K.; Sahu, P.K.; Seedial, N.; Seecharan, G.; Seepersad, A.; Seunarine, M.; Sieunarine, S.; Seymour, K.; Simboo, S.; Singh, A.; et al. An exploratory study of quality of life and its relationship with academic performance among students in medical and other health professions. *Med. Sci.* **2020**, *8*, 23. [CrossRef] [PubMed]
5. Hafen, M.; Drake, A.S.; Elmore, R.G. Predictors of psychological well-being among veterinary medical students. *J. Vet. Med. Educ.* **2023**, *50*, e20210133. [CrossRef] [PubMed]
6. Islam, R.K.; Cobb, E.K.; McCowan, H.K.; Watson, K.; Bhattacharya, K.; Chandra, A.; Mohiuddin, W.; Gruszynski, K.; Wilkerson, A.H.; Dascanio, J.J.; et al. Exploring mental health in veterinary students: Common stressors and effective coping strategies: A narrative review. *Front. Vet. Sci.* **2025**, *12*, 1470022. [CrossRef] [PubMed]
7. World Health Organization Programme on Mental Health. *WHOQOL User Manual*; WHO: Geneva, Switzerland, 2012.
8. Jaworski, J.L.; Thompson, L.A.; Weng, H.Y. Quality of life of veterinary residents in AVMA-recognized veterinary specialty organizations using the WHOQOL-BREF instrument. *PLoS ONE* **2022**, *17*, e0268343. [CrossRef] [PubMed]

medical sciences forum

MDPI

Proceeding Paper

Rethinking Science Teaching for the 21st Century: A SWOT Analysis of a Multi-Strategic Model †

Ana Isabel Fernandes [1,*] and Margarida Miranda [1,2]

1 Egas Moniz Center for Interdisciplinary Research (CiiEM), Egas Moniz School of Health & Science, 2829-511 Monte de Caparica, Portugal; mrodrigues@egasmoniz.edu.pt
2 Coimbra Chemistry Center, Department of Chemistry, University of Coimbra, 3004-535 Coimbra, Portugal
* Correspondence: aifernandes@egasmoniz.edu.pt
† Presented at the 7th CiiEM International Congress 2025—Empowering One Health to Reduce Social Vulnerabilities, Caparica, Portugal, 2–4 July 2025.

Abstract: This work presents the Integrated Multi-Strategy Teaching (IMST) model, developed for science education to enhance autonomy, engagement, and professional competencies. Applied in a pharmacy course, IMST combines flipped classrooms, peer assessment, and scenario-based learning. A SWOT analysis based on student and faculty feedback highlights strengths in skill development and practical relevance, while noting challenges such as workload and classroom constraints. The results support the effectiveness of IMST and suggest improvements to promote broader acceptance and sustainability.

Keywords: active learning; science education; pedagogical innovation; student-centred learning; SWOT analysis

1. Introduction

The rapid evolution of scientific knowledge, coupled with the complexity of professional demands in science-related fields, calls for innovative pedagogical approaches that move beyond traditional, lecture-based instruction. In science education, there is a growing emphasis on fostering deep learning, critical thinking, autonomy, and transferable skills essential for lifelong learning and adaptability [1,2]. Contemporary educational paradigms advocate for student-centred methodologies that promote active participation and engagement, such as flipped classrooms, guided self-study, peer evaluation, and scenario-based learning [3–5].

The Integrated Multi-Strategy Teaching in Science (IMTS) approach responds to these imperatives by blending diverse evidence-based strategies into a cohesive model. It has been developed, systematically applied, and improved in the pharmaceutical context, specifically of Drug Delivery and Targeting, in the last decade. It emphasizes structured autonomy, collaborative problem solving, and reflective learning, leveraging digital tools, for blended learning and continuous assessment. This pedagogical model aims not only to enhance knowledge acquisition but also to cultivate professional competencies aligned with the needs of 21st-century science graduates [5,6].

This paper summarizes the IMTS practice and presents a SWOT analysis of the methodology as applied in a university-level science course. It explores its strengths, weaknesses, opportunities, and threats, based on student outcomes and engagement levels, and the reflective input of the two faculty members involved in its development and application. The analysis explores the benefits and limitations of the approach, as well as its potential for scaling and institutional integration across academic contexts.

2. Materials and Methods

The IMST model aligns with contemporary educational trends that emphasize maximum learning with minimum teaching, structured around three core pillars: knowledge, skills, and attitudes. To foster active student engagement, a variety of strategies (e.g., flipped classes, role-playing, group work, peer assessment) are implemented during theoretical-practical sessions. The learning process typically unfolds in three phases; the key elements considered at each stage to increase effectiveness and commitment are presented:

2.1. Pre-Class

Students engage with research materials and self-study, supported by curated content. Guidelines for the weekly activities to be completed before, during, and after each class are clearly presented on Moodle platform (https://moodle.egasmoniz.edu.pt/). Content that is scientifically sound, up-to-date, and aligned with the course objectives is selected, highlighting current scientific trends and prioritizing literature reviews for a comprehensive perspective. Incorporation of examples of the professor's own work fosters interest, engagement, and relevance. Strict adherence to deadlines is enforced to promote accountability and a sense of responsibility among students.

2.2. In-Class

Interactive activities such as bibliographic search, content selection and management; ethical and responsible use of artificial intelligence (AI); production of written materials with or without oral presentation; intra- and/or inter-group discussion; problem-solving tasks or role-playing, ensure active participation. The class begins with a brief contextualisation of the activity and verification of whether autonomous preparatory work has been completed and finishes by consolidating the content, clearly and concisely summarizing key takeaways and their relevance or impact. The time allocated to each task is carefully managed to maintain focus and efficiency. Themes, media format of presentations (e.g., report, abstract, poster, oral), and communication contexts (e.g., patient, doctor, scientific meeting), are varied while also employing diverse pedagogical approaches to enhance engagement and learning.

2.3. Post-Class

To reinforce learning, students are invited to reflect on the activity and engage with curated content (e.g., short videos) or to evaluate and provide feedback on peers' work, as applicable. Credible, up-to-date multimedia resources directly aligned with the lesson topic are selected to reinforce and deepen understanding. Moodle Workshop tool is used to conduct individual, randomized peer evaluations, guided by a structured assessment grid developed by the professor to ensure fairness and consistency.

The level of complexity and autonomy required from students increases progressively throughout the course, culminating in a final group assignment. This task involves the production of an abstract and a scientific poster, which are gradually developed and refined in class with the professor's guidance.

Assessment is multi-faceted and includes written components, oral presentations—delivered both in class and at a Students' Scientific Meeting—as well as an individual discussion of the work. Evaluation is carried out by both the professor and peers, fostering accountability and reflective learning. An Objective Structured Clinical/Practical Exam (OSCPE) is applied at the end of the course as a skills assessment methodology [7].

An online survey, featuring a 16-item questionnaire with a continuous 0–10 scale, was conducted using Mentimeter (https://www.mentimeter.com/); voting outputs were invisible to participants. It targeted fourth-year pharmacy students (2024–2025; $n = 64$) at the end of the "Advanced Therapeutic Systems" course, which implemented the IMST model. The survey was applied prior to the final evaluation to reduce the impact that a less favourable mark might introduce. The questionnaire assessed students' perceptions of course structure and organization, the perceived validity and reliability of the practice, and comparisons between the IMST approach and traditional lecture-based teaching. Open-ended questions gathered qualitative feedback on strengths, weaknesses, and suggestions for improvement. Additionally, professors, independently and before treating student data to avoid bias, reflected on application of the model and student performance. A SWOT analysis was used to compare student responses and professor insights, and identify opportunities for improvement.

3. Results and Discussion

The students' perspective on the IMST model, based on an online survey (96.9% response rate), is summarized in Figure 1. Overall, the practice was well-received, with students reporting clear gains in key academic and professional skills. The results underscore the method's effectiveness in promoting autonomy, active engagement, and preparedness for professional challenges—core objectives of the IMST approach. Areas of moderate satisfaction point to opportunities for enhancing the perceived accessibility and motivational impact of learning. Notably, the highest rating was given to the increased preparation time required, reflecting a significant workload compared to traditional methods, probably explaining the moderate enjoyment as a learning strategy. Conversely, the lowest score—related to enthusiasm for study—suggests that while students valued the method, it did not always translate into greater personal motivation or emotional engagement. In open-ended responses, many students suggested carrying out most of the work during class time (22.6%), interspersing preparatory and presentation sessions (6.5%), and extending deadlines for coursework and peer evaluation (4.8%). Only one student expressed a preference for traditional classes, due to the reduced effort, a greater reliance on the professor's explanations, and concerns over the fairness of peer review.

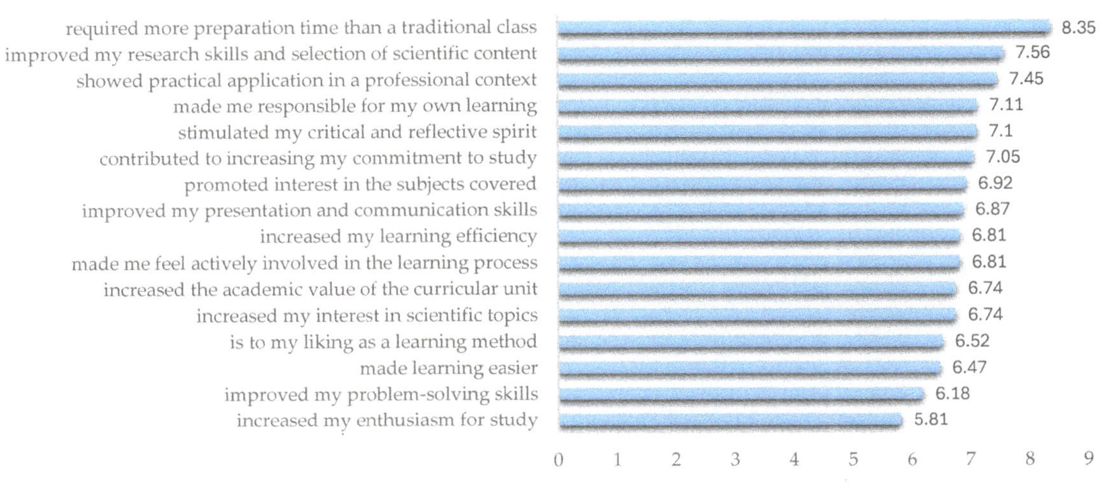

Figure 1. Student satisfaction with the IMST model in the 2024–2025 academic year.

A combined SWOT summary comparing professors' and students' perspectives regarding their experiences with the IMTS practice is given in Table 1. The pedagogical value of the model in the development of transversal and academic skills such as research, communication, and critical thinking is also recognized by professors. However, weaknesses are evident in the method's high time demands and implementation challenges—especially for students lacking autonomy or English language proficiency. Professors highlighted the logistical burden of applying IMST, including preparation and grading time, managing peer assessment, and limited classroom adaptability. Some students also failed to complete post-class tasks, weakening the learning cycle.

Table 1. Combined SWOT analysis integrating the perspectives of students **[S]**, professors **[P]** or both students and professors **[SP]**, highlighting commonalities and contrasts.

Strengths (S)	Weaknesses (W)
[S] Felt more actively involved in learning (6.81) and more responsible for their learning (7.11); **[S]** Reported gains in research (7.56), presentation and communication (6.87) skills; **[S]** Perceived practical relevance of the model (7.45); **[S]** Stated promoted learning efficiency (6.81) and interest in the subject (6.92); **[S]** IMTS stimulates critical thinking (7.10), interest in scientific topics (6.74), and commitment (7.05). —••— **[P]** Students are required to take a proactive approach to achieve the specific goals of each class; **[P]** Lessons are dynamic and diversified due to the varied teaching–learning methodologies and subjects; **[P]** Peer evaluation gives [S] a clearer understanding of their own performance, highlights areas of improvement; **[P]** Increase in transversal competencies (e.g., stress management, teamwork, communication in various contexts); **[P]** Unique group projects enrich overall learning/discussion; **[P]** IMTS fosters curricular integration and real-life simulation through final OSCPE exam.	**[S]** Found the method demanding in terms of time (8.35), with moderate enjoyment (6.52) and enthusiasm (5.81); **[S]** Moderately improved problem-solving skills (6.52) and learning ease (6.47). —••— **[P]** High workload due to preparation, marking, and feedback delivery; **[P]** Limited time in class for deep exploration and individual feedback; **[P]** Some students miss post-class tasks, leading to incomplete learning cycles; **[P]** Difficulties managing large groups and tracking peer evaluations on Moodle; **[P]** Students with poor English or lack of autonomy struggle to follow class structure; **[P]** Rigid schedules and physical classroom limitations hinder collaboration and responsiveness; **[P]** Lack of consistent post-class engagement and challenges to use OSCPE as a learning strategy due to late application (end of semester).
Opportunities (O)	**Threats (T)**
[P] Good Pedagogical Practice (awarded in 2024) offers institutional credibility and dissemination potential; **[P]** Encourage AI use for problem-solving, real-world task alignment and work opportunities; **[P]** Use high-impact elements (research, relevance) as drivers of engagement; **[P]** Adaptable to various curricula; transferable across disciplines. —••— **[SP]** Include motivation strategies (e.g., gamification); **[SP]** Feedback-driven improvements and flexible evaluation models to promote continuous refinement.	**[P]** High workload perception may reduce engagement or increase stress; **[P]** Risk of inequity if autonomy levels overwhelm less prepared students; **[P]** Unsuitable for students resistant to active learning or lacking self-discipline; **[P]** Non-native [S] may disengage due to language barriers; **[P]** Student absences and disengagement negatively affect group dynamics and outcomes; **[P]** Overreliance on AI without critical thinking can lead to unstructured or superficial learning; **[P]** Risk of professor burnout due to intense demands and limited support infrastructure; **[P]** Current peer-assessment tools (Moodle) lack transparency and efficiency for formative use.

There are clear opportunities to further refine the model by leveraging its recognition as an award-winning practice, integrating motivational strategies like gamification, and expanding its transdisciplinary reach. The strategic use of AI and continuous feedback loops also present growth paths. Nonetheless, significant threats remain, such as resistance to non-traditional methods, inequities in student readiness, and professor burnout risk due to limited support. Inadequate digital tools and classroom infrastructure further limit scalability and long-term sustainability.

4. Conclusions

The IMST model effectively cultivates active learning, professional competencies, and curricular integration. While students and professors alike recognize its educational value, its sustainability depends on addressing structural, logistical, and motivational barriers. Balancing innovation with realistic workload expectations and inclusive design is key to broadening its acceptance and impact across diverse learning environments.

Author Contributions: Conceptualization, methodology, formal analysis and data curation, writing, review and editing, A.I.F.; methodology, review and editing, M.M. All authors have read and agreed to the published version of the manuscript.

Funding: A.I.F. and M.M. thank FCT/MCTES for the financial support to CiiEM (10.54499/UIDB/04585/2020) through national funds.

Institutional Review Board Statement: As part of the educational continuous improvement strategy, no sensitive data were collected, and formal ethical approval was waived.

Informed Consent Statement: Participation was voluntary, anonymous, and consented.

Data Availability Statement: The data presented in this study are available on request.

Acknowledgments: The authors gratefully acknowledge the fourth-year pharmacy students that over the years have willingly engaged in this pedagogical experience and provided input for continuous improvement.

Conflicts of Interest: The authors declare no conflicts of interest.

References

1. Biggs, J.; Tang, C.; Kennedy, G. *Teaching for Quality Learning at University*, 5th ed.; Open University Press—McGraw Hill: Buckingham, UK, 2022; ISBN 9780335250820.
2. Prince, M. Does active learning work? A review of the research. *J. Eng. Educ.* **2004**, *93*, 223–231. [CrossRef]
3. Bergmann, J.; Sams, A. *Flip Your Classroom: Reach Every Student in Every Class Every Day*; International Society for Technology in Education: Eugene, OR, USA, 2023; ISBN 9781564849861.
4. Nicol, D.J.; Macfarlane-Dick, D. Formative assessment and self-regulated learning: A model and seven principles of good feedback practice. *Stud. High. Educ.* **2006**, *31*, 199–218. [CrossRef]
5. Freeman, S.; Eddy, S.L.; McDonough, M.; Smith, M.K.; Okoroafor, N.; Jordt, H.; Wenderoth, M.P. Active learning increases student performance in science, engineering, and mathematics. *Proc. Natl. Acad. Sci. USA* **2014**, *111*, 8410–8415. [CrossRef] [PubMed]
6. OECD. *The Future of Education and Skills: Education 2030*; OECD Publishing, Ed.; Organisation for Economic Co-Operation and Development: Paris, France, 2018.
7. Cavaco-Silva, P.; Ribeiro, A.C.; Figueiredo, A.; Guerreiro, D.; Oliveira-Torres, E.; Costa, I.M.; Couvaneiro, J.; Aguiar, J.P.; Inez, R.; Branco, V.; et al. *Objective Structured Clinical/Practical Examination (OSC/PE) in Pharmaceutical Sciences Education—A Pilot Study*; Ramos, F., Ed.; Ordem dos Farmacêuticos, SRP: Porto, Portugal, 2023.

medical sciences forum

MDPI

Proceeding Paper

Attitudes Toward Community Service Among Higher Health Sciences Students †

Sónia Vicente [1,*], Ângela Maria Pereira [1,2], Ana Cristina Vidal [1,2] and Cláudia Maria Costa [3]

1 Egas Moniz Center for Interdisciplinary Research (CiiEM), Egas Moniz School of Health & Science, Caparica, 2829-511 Almada, Portugal; apereira@egasmoniz.edu.pt (Â.M.P.); avidal@egasmoniz.edu.pt (A.C.V.)

2 Hospital Garcia de Orta, Unidade Local de Saúde Almada Seixal, 2805-267 Almada, Portugal

3 Physiotherapy Department, Escola Superior de Saúde Atlântica, 2730-036 Barcarena, Portugal; ccosta@uatlantica.pt

* Correspondence: svicente@egasmoniz.edu.pt

† Presented at the 7th CiiEM International Congress 2025—Empowering One Health to Reduce Social Vulnerabilities, Caparica, Portugal, 2–4 July 2025.

Abstract: University Social Responsibility (USR) integrates academic goals with ethics, civic engagement, and sustainability. This study assessed community service attitudes among 529 higher health sciences students using the Portuguese Community Service Attitudes Scale. Although 52.9% reported prior volunteer experience, 75.2% had not participated in community service during university. An association was found between academic programme and prior involvement, particularly among Dental Medicine and Physiotherapy students. While no sex differences were observed, programme-specific trends suggest that practical training fosters stronger civic responsibility. Integrating structured, discipline-specific community service into curricula may enhance civic identity and better align education with sustainable development goals.

Keywords: university social responsibility; community service; higher education; student attitudes; civic engagement

1. Introduction

Higher education institutions (HEIs) are increasingly challenged to extend their traditional roles beyond teaching and research to address broader societal concerns [1,2]. In Portugal, a growing emphasis on the social dimension and community engagement of HEIs has emerged as a central concern. The Observatory for Social Responsibility and Higher Education Institutions (ORSIES) in Portugal has developed a strategic vision for social responsibility in higher education and established a framework of social responsibility indicators to support self-assessment and continuous improvement among HEIs [3]. Within this context, USR is seen as a crucial commitment, aiming to prepare students not only for their future professional careers but also as critical and engaged citizens [1,3]. This is particularly relevant in the field of health sciences, where higher health schools are increasingly expected to align their education, research, and service activities with the priority health needs of the communities they serve [4]. Despite the recognised potential of USR projects to foster active citizenship and transversal competencies among students [1], there remains a scarcity of studies exploring students' direct conceptions of and engagement with USR, particularly concerning the impact of their involvement in such initiatives [3]. For instance, a study involving Portuguese universities revealed that nearly half of the surveyed students had not heard of USR in their university, pointing to the need for clearer communication on the topic [1]. Furthermore, although there has been overall progress in the implementation of social responsibility indicators in Portuguese HEIs, some areas still show persistently low levels of formalisation and implementation [3]. Despite efforts, a deeper understanding, greater formalisation, and broader stakeholder involvement in the concept of USR remain necessary across Portuguese HEIs [3]. Furthermore, a significant gap persists in the literature regarding robust and generalised measures for assessing the effectiveness of community service programmes, particularly in relation to the attitudes students develop [5]. Understanding these attitudes is vital, as today's students will be future professionals and citizens responsible for addressing societal challenges [6]. The aim of this study is to evaluate the attitudes of higher health students at Egas Moniz School of Health & Sciences toward community service within higher sciences education.

2. Materials and Methods

2.1. Study Design

A descriptive, observational, and cross-sectional design was used.

2.2. Participants

This study included 529 university health students at Egas Moniz School of Health & Sciences, recruited using a convenience sampling method. The inclusion criteria were students enrolled in a health sciences course at a Portuguese higher education institution, aged over eighteen years, able to understand Portuguese, and able to provide informed consent. All incomplete questionnaires were excluded.

2.3. Instrument, Data Collection, and Management

Participation in the study was voluntary and anonymous, with informed consent obtained from all participants. The research was approved by the Egas Moniz Ethics Committee (Process No. 1106, 30 June 2022). Data was collected via Google Forms from March to July 2024. The questionnaire was disseminated via institutional email, with the support of colleagues collaborating on the project, as well as through formal and informal student networks. Participants completed a 15 min questionnaire that included the Portuguese version of the Community Service Attitudes Scale (CSAS), along with demographic (age and sex), academic (course, studies' year, and level of study), and community service experience data, following previous studies [4,7]. The CSAS is a 46-item tool based on Schwartz's model of altruistic helping behaviour, organised into four stages and ten dimensions: *Perception of the Need to Respond* (Awareness, Actions, Ability, and Connectedness); *Moral Obligation to Respond* (Norms and Empathy); *Reassessment* (Costs, Benefits, and Seriousness); and *Engagement in Helping Behaviour* (Intention to Become Involved). Responses are rated on a 7-point Likert scale [8,9]. Dimension scores are calculated by summing the item responses. The Portuguese version showed strong psychometric properties, with Cronbach's alpha values above 0.80 across all dimensions (total score $\alpha = 0.97$; subscales $\alpha = 0.88$–0.95) and high test–retest reliability (ICC = 0.96 for total score; 0.86–0.94 for subscales) [10].

2.4. Statistical Analysis

Data distribution was analysed using the Kolmogorov–Smirnov test. As the assumptions for normality were not met, non-parametric tests were applied. A descriptive analysis was performed to characterise the sample. Chi-square (for ordinal variables) and Mann–Whitney U (for continuous variables) tests were used to analyse potential differences and compare dimensions of the community attitudes scale between two groups (e.g., sex and previous community work experience). The Kruskal–Wallis test with the Bonferroni correction was applied for comparisons involving multiple groups (e.g., degree programme and academic year). The level of significance was set at $p < 0.05$. All tests were performed using SPSS for Windows, version 29.

3. Results

A total of 529 students responded (mean age 20.7 ± 4.5 years; 74.5% female). Most were bachelor's students (87.5%), followed by master's students (12.3%) and PhD students (0.2%). The majority of respondents (55.5%) were in their second or third year of a bachelor's programme. Participants represented a range of health science disciplines: Dental Medicine (DM) (51.6%), Physiotherapy (PT) (27.8%), Psychology (Psy) (10.2%), Pharmacy (Pharm) (5.3%), Nursing (2.5%), and Biomedical Laboratory Sciences (BMLC) (2.6%). While 52.9% reported previous volunteer experience, 75.2% indicated no participation in community service since the beginning of their academic studies, indicating a drop in civic engagement during university years. Only 4.3% reported weekly participation. Chi-square analysis revealed a significant association between academic programme and prior community experience ($p < 0.001$), particularly among DM and PT. Although no significant sex differences were observed, programme-specific differences did emerge. Pharmacy students scored significantly higher in Ability (vs. BMLC: $p = 0.006$; DM: $p = 0.022$; PT: $p = 0.030$), Connectedness (vs. PT: $p = 0.019$; Psy: $p = 0.044$), and Norms (vs. BMLC: $p = 0.007$; Psy: $p = 0.006$; PT: $p = 0.004$; DM: $p = 0.016$). Dental Medicine students scored higher in Perceived Benefits (vs. PT: $p = 0.040$). A marginal association was found between year of study and community involvement ($p = 0.064$), suggesting a trend toward greater engagement in later years or clinical phases, though this was not statistically significant. These findings suggest that students from Pharmacy and Dental Medicine perceive themselves as more capable, aligned with social norms, and connected in relation to community involvement, compared to students from other programmes.

4. Discussion

This study identified programme-specific differences in university students' attitudes toward community service and social responsibility, reinforcing findings from the previous literature emphasising the importance of course context and institutional culture in shaping civic engagement among higher education students [1,11]. Despite a higher proportion of female participants—reflecting national higher education trends in Portugal [12]—no significant sex (biological attribute) differences in attitudes toward community service were found. This finding aligns with earlier studies showing a higher number of female participants in USR and volunteering research [13]. However, the literature offers mixed insights on how sex affects perceptions of USR. While some studies found no significant sex differences [1,6], others suggest that female students often score higher on the CSAS [8]. Our results indicate that sex may not be a decisive factor for general perceptions of social responsibility, although it might influence the level of critical engagement or benevolence exacted in assessing university practices. A key finding was the link between academic programme and prior community engagement, with DM and PT students more likely to report previous experience. This supports the idea that certain curricula, especially in "helping" professions, foster stronger attitudes toward social responsibility [8]. While there is no direct evidence explaining why these two fields stood out, the presence of clinical facilities at the university likely plays a role by enabling early interactions with patients. Previous studies have shown that programmes with strong community ties and practical applications tend to encourage more meaningful social engagement [1]. There were notable differences in students' attitudes toward community service across academic programmes. Pharmacy students scored higher in *Ability*, *Connectedness*, and *Norms*, indicating stronger confidence, civic values, and social ties. DM students perceived greater *Benefits* than PT students. These differences likely reflect variations in curriculum focus, professional identity development, and early exposure to social roles. The higher scores among Pharmacy students may be linked to most respondents being in later years of education, with a clearer sense of their community role. This supports prior findings that disciplinary context and programme stage influence civic attitudes, especially in fields tied closely to public service [1,14].

5. Conclusions

This study highlights promising indicators of student engagement with community service and social responsibility within our university context. The findings suggest that the current institutional initiatives are already fostering awareness and positive attitudes among students. However, the variation observed across academic programmes points to the need for a more cohesive and integrated approach. Strengthening the incorporation of University Social Responsibility (USR) into curricula—through experiential learning, critical reflection, and interdisciplinary opportunities—can further support the development of socially engaged and ethically responsible professionals. Building on existing efforts, HEIs will be well-positioned to strengthen their leadership role in driving social transformation and achieving a meaningful, sustained community impact. Future studies should aim to include a larger and more balanced sample and consider comparisons with other higher education institutions to enhance the generalisability and depth of these findings.

Author Contributions: Conceptualisation: S.V., A.C.V., and C.M.C.; methodology: S.V., software: S.V., data curation: S.V., Formal analysis: Â.M.P., Writing—original draft: S.V., Writing—review and editing: C.M.C. and Â.M.P., supervision: C.M.C. All authors have read and agreed to the published version of the manuscript.

Funding: This research received no external funding.

Institutional Review Board Statement: This study was conducted in accordance with the Declaration of Helsinki and approved by the Egas Moniz Ethics Committee (Process No. 1106 of 30 June 2022).

Informed Consent Statement: Informed consent was obtained from all subjects involved in this study.

Data Availability Statement: The data will be made available by the corresponding author upon request.

Acknowledgments: The authors acknowledge the support of the Board of Directors and Course Coordinators as well as the student participation.

Conflicts of Interest: The authors declare no conflicts of interest.

References

1. Coelho, M.; Menezes, I. University Social Responsibility, Service Learning, and Students' Personal, Professional, and Civic Education. *Front. Psychol.* **2021**, *12*, 617300. [CrossRef] [PubMed]
2. Manzano-Sánchez, D.; Gómez-Marmol, A.; Jiménez-Parra, J.F.; Bohórquez, I.G.; Valero-Valenzuela, A. Motivational profiles and their relationship with responsibility, school social climate and resilience in high school students. *PLoS ONE* **2021**, *16*, e0256293. [CrossRef] [PubMed]
3. Observatório da Responsabilidade Social e Instituições de Ensino Superior (ORSIES). *Relatório Global ORSIES 2021–2022*; ORSIES: Lisboa, Portugal, 2022; Available online: https://www.orsies.forum.pt (accessed on 15 May 2025).
4. Pearson, D.; Walpole, S.; Barna, S. Challenges to professionalism: Social accountability and global environmental change. *Med. Teach.* **2015**, *37*, 825–830. [CrossRef] [PubMed]
5. Perry, B.; Osbaldiston, R.; Henning, J. Tests of the Validity and Reliability of the Community Service Attitudes Scale. *J. Coll. Stud. Dev.* **2014**, *55*, 726–731. [CrossRef]

6. Morales-Gualdrón, S.T.; La Rotta, D.A.; Vergara, J.A.; Ardila, J.M.; Bañol, C.H. Corporate Social Responsibility Practices of Colombian Companies as Perceived by Industrial Engineering Students. *Sci. Eng. Ethics* **2020**, *26*, 3183–3215. [CrossRef] [PubMed]
7. Phalwane, M.G.; Postma, T.C.; Ayo-Yusuf, O.A. Piloting the Community Service Attitudes Scale in a South African context with matching qualitative data. *S. Afr. Dent. J.* **2016**, *71*, 460–466.
8. Shiarella, A.H.; Mccarthy, A.M.; Tucker, M.L. Development and Construct Validity of Scores on the Community Service Attitudes Scale. *Educ. Psychol. Meas.* **2000**, *60*, 286–300. [CrossRef]
9. Simmer-Beck, M.; Gadbury-Amyot, C.; Williams, K.B.; Keselyak, N.T.; Branson, B.; Mitchell, T.V. Measuring the short-term effects of incorporating academic service learning throughout a dental hygiene curriculum. *Int. J. Dent. Hyg.* **2013**, *11*, 260–266. [CrossRef] [PubMed]
10. Vicente, S.; Pereira, A.M.; Vidal, A.C.; Costa, C.M. Cross cultural adaptation and validation of the Portuguese version of the Community Service Attitudes scale. *Educ. Assess. Eval. Account.* 2024; *submitted*.
11. Govindaraj, Y.; Pandiyaraj, G. Social responsibility and leadership behaviour among higher educational students in the 21st century. *AJUE* **2022**, *18*, 1119–1129.
12. PORDATA. Available online: https://www.pordata.pt/pt/search?search=percentagem%20estudantes%20do%20ensino%20superior%20por%20sexo (accessed on 20 June 2025).
13. Berei, E.B. The social responsibility among higher education students. *Educ. Sci.* **2020**, *10*, 66. [CrossRef]
14. Gomez, I.; Fowkes, V.; Price, I. Teaching community engagement for health professions students in underserved areas. *Discov. Educ.* **2024**, *3*, 244. [CrossRef]

medical sciences forum

MDPI

Proceeding Paper

The PROMOTE Project in Portugal: Rethinking Reintegration Through the National Adaptation Workshop †

Iris Almeida [1,*], Ana Nascimento David [2], Ana Rita Lourenço [3], Guilherme Sena [4], Maria Alexandra Garrafão [3] and Ricardo Ventura Baúto [1]

1 Laboratory of Forensic and Psychological Sciences Egas Moniz, CiiEM—Egas Moniz Center for Interdisciplinary Research, Egas Moniz School of Health and Science, Caparica, 2829-511 Almada, Portugal; rbauto@egasmoniz.edu.pt

2 IPS Innovative Prison Systems, Avenida Doutor Mário Moutinho 33-A (Office 5), 1400-136 Lisbon, Portugal; ana.nascimento@prisonsystems.eu

3 APROXIMAR, Cooperativa de Solidariedade Social, CRL, Rua do Paraíso, Loja n.° 2, 2610-136 Alfragide, Portugal; rita.alves@aproximar.pt (A.R.L.); alexandra.garrafao@aproximar.pt (M.A.G.)

4 Egas Moniz School of Health and Science, Caparica, 2829-511 Almada, Portugal; guisenacosta@gmail.com

* Correspondence: ialmeida@egasmoniz.edu.pt

† Presented at the 7th CiiEM International Congress 2025—Empowering One Health to Reduce Social Vulnerabilities, Caparica, Portugal, 2–4 July 2025.

Abstract: This study explores the implementation of competency-based professional development for correctional staff through the DACUM (Developing A Curriculum) methodology. A National Adaptation Workshop in Portugal engaged professionals from multiple sectors—psychologists, social workers, educators, prison officers, re-education and reintegration technicians—to validate occupational profiles and training needs. Thematic analysis revealed gaps between required and available training, especially in conflict management, mental health, and interdisciplinary collaboration. Key findings show strong support for participatory, practice-informed training, provided it is contextually adapted and accessible. The results underscore the practical need for flexible, modular training frameworks in correctional settings, offering implications for policy and staff retention strategies.

Keywords: PROMOTE; training; correctional services; professional profiles

1. Introduction

The prison environment is marked by institutional rigidity, social vulnerability, and psychosocial tension. Professionals operating within such settings, including psychologists, educators, reintegration officers, and correctional staff, face multifaceted challenges that extend far beyond custodial duties. Their roles increasingly involve psychosocial intervention, educational support, and the facilitation of inmates' reintegration into society [1,2]. However, despite the complexity of their mandates, these professionals often lack access to continuous, specialised training tailored to the specificities of penal institutions [3].

Contemporary correctional systems across Europe emphasise rehabilitation and social reintegration as key objectives of incarceration. This transformation implies a shift from punitive to human service roles, in which correctional staff are required not only to maintain institutional order but also to foster behavioural change and promote personal development among inmates [4–6]. In a study by Miklóski [1], it became apparent that the Hungarian experience illustrates this shift, with structured training models aiming to enhance competencies such as communication, conflict resolution, emotional regulation, and intercultural sensitivity.

 https://doi.org/10.3390/msf2025037023

Empirical findings indicate a significant gap between the competencies required in prison work and the training professionals receive. For example, a study involving staff working with juvenile offenders revealed widespread self-reported inadequacy in dealing with aggression, addictions, and sexual offences—critical areas in prison dynamics [3]. Similar concerns emerge in the Hungarian penitentiary context, where short initial training periods and high staff turnover threaten the quality of institutional functioning [1].

In response, the literature advocates competency-based and experiential learning models that emphasise practical knowledge, psychological resilience, and reflective practice. Progressive training methods—such as role play, case study analysis, group work, and supervision—are highlighted as more effective than traditional lecture-based approaches in fostering autonomous, adaptable, and ethically grounded professionals [7,8]. Furthermore, mentoring systems and career development strategies are essential for staff retention and professional identity consolidation [9].

The PROMOTE Project (Promoting Integrated Professional Development for Prison Practitioners), co-funded by the European Union (PROMOTE—101144006—ERASMUS-EDU-2023-PEX-COVE), aligns with these recommendations by proposing the implementation of collaborative training groups for professionals working with incarcerated populations. These groups aim to provide a structured environment for skill development, knowledge exchange, and psychosocial support, thereby enhancing the quality and ethical grounding of professional interventions. Ultimately, this initiative seeks to contribute to a correctional culture that balances institutional security with human dignity and rehabilitation. It focuses on identifying professional profiles, required competencies, and training needs.

2. Materials and Methods

2.1. *Methodological Framework: DACUM Approach*

This study adopted a participatory, competence-based methodology (DACUM—Developing A Curriculum) to identify key tasks, skills, and training needs of professionals working with incarcerated individuals [10]. The research was conducted within the scope of the PROMOTE project through a National Adaptation Workshop led by the Egas Moniz School of Health and Science (Work Package 2—WP2).

2.2. *Workshop Structure and Participant Profile*

The workshop brought together 11 professionals from diverse correctional roles—prison officers, psychologists, re-education technicians, and reintegration officers. Through structured group exercises, participants validated occupational profiles using DACUM checklists informed by prior surveys, interviews, and policy analyses.

Workshop activities included a briefing on the DACUM methodology, small group discussions around occupational roles, and a consensus-building process to assess the relevance of proposed competencies and training needs.

2.3. *Qualitative Analysis Procedures*

All workshop contributions—written notes, verbal exchanges, and group summaries—were documented and subjected to thematic analysis. An initial coding phase was conducted by a single researcher, who identified recurring patterns and divergent viewpoints. To improve the rigour and credibility of the analysis, the emerging themes were then reviewed by the project team through a collaborative validation session. This helped ensure interpretive consensus and alignment with the local institutional context.

3. Results and Discussion

3.1. Validation of Professional Profiles

The results of the National Adaptation Workshop reinforce the relevance of a competency-based, practitioner-informed approach to professional development in correctional settings. Participants from diverse occupational backgrounds confirmed the general validity of the PROMOTE profiles, while also highlighting critical nuances requiring contextual adjustment, as demonstrated in Table 1. All occupational groups provided structured feedback across several key dimensions: Duties and Tasks, Competencies, Attitudes, Knowledge, and Training Needs.

Table 1. Validation of professional profiles.

Professional Profile	Section	Validation Level	Non-Validated Items
Prison Guard	DT	Partial	1: (a); 3: (b), (e), (g), (i); 4: (a), (c); 5: all items (except Head of Corps: (b), (h), (i))
	C	High, with notes	13, 21, 24 (contextual limits and responsibilities)
	A	Full	None
	K	High	None (note: not formally required)
	TN	Full, with caveats	None (note: training not available)
Psychologist	DT	High	2. (g), 2. (h); 7. (a), (b), (c)
	C	Full	None
	A	Full	None (note: limits to confidentiality in item 10)
	K	Full	None (suggested: basic life support)
	TN	High	1, 16
Re-education Technician	DT	High	2. (o)
	C	Full	None
	A	High	10
	K	Full	None
	TN	Full	None
Reintegration Technician	DT	Moderate	1. (f), (g); 2. (f); 3. (e), (f), (g); 4. (a), (b), (c); 5. (b), (c), (i); 9. (f), (h), (i), (m), (p), (q)
	C	Full	None
	A	Full	None (repetition in 1 and 8 and 3 and 12)
	K	High	4, 19
	TN	High	22, 23

Note: Full—fully validated; High—largely validated with minor reservations; Moderate—partially validated; Partial—some aspects validated; Not Validated—rejected.

3.1.1. Duties and Tasks (DT)

Participants from all professional groups shared reflections to refine and contextualise role expectations. Clarifying responsibilities was a recurring theme. Re-education technicians noted overlaps with psychologists in therapeutic tasks, stressing these belong to licensed mental health professionals. Reflections across professional groups revealed the need to clarify role expectations [e.g., "It is necessary to restructure the legislation (. . .) our professional actions are limited (. . .)."]. These observations echo prior studies on the importance of role clarity in complex institutional environments [1,3].

3.1.2. Competencies (C)

Feedback from prison guards and psychologists centred on functional boundaries and the necessity of role-specific differentiation. Guards underlined their limited authority in disciplinary decisions, which are formally reserved for institutional boards. One participant remarked: "Prison guards are only responsible for the application of disciplinary (. . .)" Psychologists advocated for an expanded role in mental health policy and inter-institutional coordination, reinforcing the imperative for adaptive competency on future frameworks [1].

3.1.3. Attitudes (A)

The dimension of professional attitudes was widely endorsed, with guards and technicians emphasising the ethical handling of security-related information. A guard made the following observation: "Our duty obligates us to communicate situations that may present a risk to the order and safety of the prison." Balancing firmness with rehabilitation was seen as requiring judgement, reflecting the emotional and ethical demands of correctional work [2].

3.1.4. Knowledge (K)

Comments in this area indicated a disparity between formally required knowledge and actual practice, particularly among prison guards and reintegration professionals. A participant made the following remark: "The majority of these items are not a requirement for the function and this knowledge is only acquired through the initiative of each individual prison guard." Psychologists proposed basic life support as a relevant knowledge area. These insights support earlier arguments that training frameworks must move beyond prescriptive curricula and incorporate experiential, practice-informed learning [7].

3.1.5. Training Needs (TN)

Although the training needs were largely endorsed, participants reported significant gaps in training availability and access. Also, the work overload and understaffing make it difficult to attend training. Prison guards noted that most recommended training is not offered. Additionally, professionals across groups suggested integrating emerging topics, such as restorative justice and applied statistics for psychologists, or interpersonal skills and conflict management for prison guards [e.g., "The training proposed is relevant, but not accessible. We need training that supports our actual challenges (. . .)."].

3.2. *Applicability of Best Practices*

Participants broadly acknowledged the relevance of international training models but emphasised the need for contextual adaptation, especially concerning legal frameworks and institutional infrastructure. Table 2 outlines the perceived applicability of proposed practices by professional group. While most practices were deemed relevant, their feasibility was often contingent on structural and legal conditions.

Table 2. Applicability of proposed practices by professional group.

Professional Group	Practice 1	Practice 2	Practice 3	Practice 4	Practice 5
Prison Guards	App	APP	APP	RA-SC	APP
Psychologists	APP-FL	APP-FL	NA	APP-T	APP-FL
Re-education Technicians	APP-CP	NA	NA	NA	APP
Reintegration Technicians	NA	NA	NA	APP	APP-IP

Note: APP = applicable; RA-SC = requires adaptation (shared cell occupancy); APP-FL = applicable with funding/licensing; APP-T = applicable for training only; APP-CP = applicable with comprehensive planning; APP-IP = applicable (in progress); NA = not applicable.

4. Conclusions

The Portuguese National Adaptation Workshop confirmed the value of participatory, competency-based approaches to professional development in correctional environments. The use of the DACUM methodology allowed for practitioner voices to shape and validate occupational profiles, enhancing contextual relevance.

Key outcomes included the need for clearer role differentiation, the misalignment between formal training provisions and institutional demands, and a call for accessible, interdisciplinary, and practice-oriented training models.

To advance these findings, future phases of the PROMOTE project should integrate flexible training modules, mentorship systems, and collaborative learning strategies. Such measures not only respond to national needs but also align with broader European efforts to humanise correctional systems through professional capacity building.

Author Contributions: Conceptualisation, I.A. and G.S.; methodology, A.N.D., A.R.L. and M.A.G.; validation, A.N.D., A.R.L. and M.A.G.; formal analysis, A.N.D.; investigation, A.N.D., A.R.L. and M.A.G.; resources, A.N.D., A.R.L. and M.A.G.; data curation, A.N.D.; writing—original draft preparation, I.A., G.S. and R.V.B.; writing—review and editing, I.A., G.S. and R.V.B.; visualisation, I.A.; supervision, I.A.; project administration, A.N.D., A.R.L. and I.A.; funding acquisition, A.N.D. and A.R.L. All authors have read and agreed to the published version of the manuscript.

Funding: The PROMOTE Project co-funded by the European Union (PROMOTE—101144006—ERASMUS-EDU-2023-PEX-COVE).

Institutional Review Board Statement: The study was conducted in accordance with the Declaration of Helsinki, and all ethical standards of scientific research were respected, as well as the General Data Protection Regulation approved by the European Union (PROMOTE—101144006).

Informed Consent Statement: All ethical issues were considered due to the sensitive nature of the detailed data, the respective informed consent and confidentiality limits.

Data Availability Statement: Data sharing not applicable because part of information derives from a European Project.

Conflicts of Interest: Author Ana Nascimento David was employed by the company IPS Innovative Prison Systems. Author Ana Rita Lourenço and Maria Alexandra Garrafão were employed by the company APROXIMAR. The remaining authors declare that the research was conducted in the absence of any commercial or financial relationships that could be construed as a potential conflict of interest.

References

1. Miklósi, M. The system of training Hungarian prison staff with a special aspect of competency development. *J. Psychol. Educ. Res.* **2023**, *31*, 113–129.
2. Liebling, A.; Price, D.; Shefer, G. *The Prison Officer*; Willan Publishing: Cullompton, UK, 2010.
3. Toma, C. Identify the needs for continuous professional training of specialists working with juvenile delinquents in order to make the intervention more effective and increase the chances of social adaptation. *J. Psychol. Educ. Res.* **2022**, *30*, 163–175. [CrossRef]
4. Giavrimis, P. The training of prison guards: The case of Greece. *Int. J. Criminol. Sociol. Theory* **2012**, *5*, 871–885.
5. King, S. Reconciling custodial and human service work: The complex role of the prison officer. *Curr. Issues Crim. Justice* **2009**, *21*, 257–272. [CrossRef]
6. Council of Europe Committee of Ministers. *The European Prison Rules*; Council of Europe: Strasbourg, France, 2006. Available online: https://rm.coe.int/european-prison-rules-978-92-871-5982-3/16806ab9ae (accessed on 18 June 2025).
7. Molnár, K.; Krémer, F. A szociális kompetenciák szerepe a mester szintű rendészeti képzésben [The role of social competences in master's level law enforcement training]. *Rendvédelmi Füzetek* **2010**, *11*, 21–32.
8. Ruzsonyi, P. Rendszerben látni, rendszerben gondolkodni: Stratégia és didaktika [Seeing in a system, thinking in a system: Strategy and didactics]. *Börtönügyi Szemle* **2018**, *37*, 77–87.

9. Büntetés-Végrehajtás Országos Parancsnoksága. Évkönyv [Yearbook]. 2021. Available online: https://bv.gov.hu/sites/default/files/BVOP_evkonyv_2021.pdf (accessed on 18 June 2025).
10. Norton, R.E. The DACUM Curriculum Development Process. In Proceedings of the Paper Presented at: International TVET Conference, Vienna, Austria, August 2004. Available online: http://www.dacumohiostate.com (accessed on 18 June 2025).

medical sciences forum

MDPI

Proceeding Paper

Robotic Gait Training in an Adolescent with Idiopathic Transverse Myelitis: A Case Report †

Maria Ana Neves *, André Lima, Gonçalo Duarte, Susana Wandschneider, Tiago Teixeira, Lia Jacobsohn, Carlos Ernesto Júnior and Isabel Batalha

Centro de Medicina de Reabilitação de Alcoitão, Rua Conde Barão, 2649-506 Alcabideche, Portugal
* Correspondence: ana.neves@scml.pt

† Presented at the 7th CiiEM International Congress 2025—Empowering One Health to Reduce Social Vulnerabilities, Caparica, Portugal, 2–4 July 2025.

Abstract: Transverse myelitis is a rare spinal cord condition that can cause severe motor, sensory, and autonomic dysfunction. This case report describes a 16-year-old male with incomplete paraplegia due to idiopathic transverse myelitis who underwent robotic-assisted gait training (RAGT) using the EKSO exoskeleton, integrated into an intensive rehabilitation programme. After one month, he showed significant improvements in gait speed, dynamic balance, effort tolerance, and trunk mobility. RAGT promoted better weight distribution and reduced compensatory patterns during ambulation. The intervention proved safe and clinically beneficial, highlighting the potential of robotic technologies as effective adjuncts in paediatric spinal cord injury rehabilitation.

Keywords: transverse myelitis; neurological rehabilitation; physiotherapy; robotic exoskeleton; gait training

1. Introduction

Transverse myelitis (TM) is a rare, rapidly progressing inflammatory disorder of the spinal cord, characterised by demyelination and resulting neurological dysfunction below the level of the lesion. It typically presents with motor weakness, sensory deficits at a defined level, and autonomic disturbances [1,2]. In paediatric populations, TM has an estimated incidence of 1 to 3 cases per million children per year, most commonly affecting those under the age of five and adolescents [2].

Walking is a key milestone in TM recovery, particularly in children, as it supports independence. Gait impairments depend on the lesion's level and severity, which affect motor control, strength, and tone in the trunk and lower limbs (LLs), which reduce participation in daily activities at home, school, and in the community [3–5].

Robotic-Assisted Gait Training (RAGT) is a promising strategy for locomotor recovery, leveraging neuroplasticity—the central nervous system's ability to reorganise structurally and functionally in response to repetitive, task-specific input. Children, with their heightened neuroplastic potential, may respond well to such interventions; however, current evidence remains limited and heterogeneous [3,5]. There are various types of RAGT depending on the level of support provided. Robotic exoskeletons were designed to assist lower limb (LL) movement and support sit-to-stand transitions and walking [4,5], supporting gait rehabilitation by enhancing propulsion, reducing body weight load, and improving proprioceptive input. Upright positioning and bilateral LL loading are critical for stimulating proprioceptors and activating spinal pathways. This sensory input—reinforced through progressive weight-bearing and hip extension—promotes sensorimotor integration. By minimising compensatory movements, exoskeleton-assisted training enhances postural control and supports upper limb balance. Additionally, it facilitates retention of functional walking patterns [2]. Furthermore, in individuals with SCI patients, has shown greater benefits than conventional therapy, improving balance, effort tolerance, strength, spasticity, and respiratory function [4,6]. It is recommended that RAGT sessions last approximately 25 min [2].

This case study aims to demonstrate, over the course of a one-month rehabilitation programme, the effectiveness of integrating a robotic exoskeleton into the physiotherapy protocol to improve gait quality and spatiotemporal parameters in paediatric patients with incomplete SCI.

2. Materials and Methods

2.1. Participant

The participant was a 16-year-old male with D8 SCI, diagnosed with idiopathic TM involving the conus medullaris, classified according to the American Spinal Injury Association Impairment Scale (AIS) as AIS B paraplegia, with a neurological level of T11. He was 4 months post-injury at the time of enrolment, 1.71 m tall, and weighed 53.6 kg. Data collection was carried out with the informed consent of the participant and his parents, including explicit authorization for the collection and disclosure of clinical information for scientific research purposes and subsequent publication.

Prior to initiating RAGT, the participant underwent a detailed clinical assessment. No limitations were observed in joint range of motion or upper limb muscle strength. However, muscular weakness was evident in the trunk and the right LL, along with a complete absence of active movement in the left LL. Sensory function was preserved above the level of T11 in the spinal cord injury and reduced below, with greater impairment observed in the left LL. From a functional standpoint, was independent in bed mobility but required assistance for positional changes, relying heavily on compensatory overuse of the right LL. The participant was able to independently assume and maintain a seated position with effective postural balance. Upright posture was achieved with assistance and the use of a knee–ankle–foot orthosis (KAFO) on the left LL, compensating for the absence of active motor control. In standing, the participant required additional support to maintain posture or perform tasks due to limited postural control. No active weight transfer was observed onto the left LL, resulting in overuse of the right hemibody during functional tasks. This was accompanied by fixation and compensatory movement patterns on the right side. Even with external support, the participant was unable to achieve single-limb stance on the left side. Ambulation was possible over short distances on flat surfaces, using two elbow crutches in combination with a KAFO. The gait pattern was markedly asymmetrical, with overuse of the right hemibody. The right stance phase was prolonged, with excessive weight transfer compensating for the difficulty in initiating left step advancement. Conversely, the left swing phase was achieved through compensatory patterns, including ipsilateral pelvic hike, quadratus lumborum activation, and elevation of the upper right trunk to enable step circumduction. The left stance phase was nearly absent, as the participant was unable to advance the hip or initiate extension, which impeded effective weight transfer and consequently led to a shortened right swing phase. Quantitative gait assessments—10-Metre Walk Test (10MWT) for gait speed, the Timed Up and Go (TUG) test for dynamic balance, the 6-Minute Walk Test (6MWT) and the Rate of Perceived Exertion (RPE) for evaluating effort tolerance and perceived exertion—along with the Berg Balance Scale (BBS) for overall balance—are presented in Table 1.

Table 1. Pre- and post-intervention spatiotemporal balance performance and gait parameters; T1: initial evaluation, T2: final evaluation, BBS: Berg Balance Scale, 10MWT: 10-Metre Walk Test, TUG: Timed Up and Go, 6MWT: 6 Minute Walk Test, RPE: Rate of Perceived Exertion.

	BBS	10MWT		TUG		6MWT			
		Time (s)	Velocity (m/s)	Time (s)	Velocity (m/s)	Distance (m)	Velocity (m/s)	Initial Perceived Exertion (RPE)	Final Perceived Exertion (RPE)
T1	14/56	22	0.45	22	0.27	163	0.45	0/10	4/10
T2	25/56	18	0.56	17	0.35	205	0.57	0/10	1/10

2.2. Rehabilitation Protocol

The participant underwent an intensive multidisciplinary rehabilitation programme in a paediatric inpatient unit, with goals integrated into a personalised plan based on recovery stage and functional needs. Physiotherapy was provided twice daily on weekdays, totalling three hours per day, by the same therapist to ensure continuity.

The physiotherapy intervention aimed to enhance functional capacity and autonomy, in accordance with current clinical guidelines for incomplete SCI. The approach was grounded in principles of neuroplasticity-based rehabilitation, incorporating meaningful, task-oriented activities. Included manual therapy and positioning, strength and endurance training, balance and mobility exercises, and functional activity training [7]. After one month of inpatient rehabilitation, RAGT sessions were introduced at a frequency of two to three times per week. Each session lasted 30 min and included the setup of the exoskeleton, tailored to the participant's physical characteristics and aligned with session goals. The intervention focused on overground gait training on a flat surface, and all sessions were conducted by two physiotherapists with specialised training in RAGT.

3. Results

Four months post-injury, Ekso was introduced to support sensorimotor integration, postural stability, and symmetrical weight distribution during gait, with a focus on improving left lower limb (LL) weight transfer, while using a KAFO. Over one month, patient completed 11 RAGT sessions (mean effective walking time: 15.64 ± 4.7 min), showing functional improvements following the combined physiotherapy and RAGT programme.

Improvements in biomechanical gait alignment were evident through clinical observation, including enhanced weight-bearing capacity on the more affected lower limb and improved sensorimotor integration. This progress enabled the patient to achieve a supported single-limb stance on the left lower limb. Although this did not yet permit the execution of specific functional tasks, it represents a positive prognostic indicator for future recovery. The structured and pre-programmed nature of RAGT facilitated safe and effective weight-shifting, allowing for more balanced lower limb loading and improved interlimb coordination to be observed. In addition, it contributed to an overall improvement in movement patterns by reducing the need for compensatory strategies. Prior to the intervention, the patient demonstrated significant difficulty bearing weight on the left LL, resulting in compensatory trunk movements to maintain gait. Post-intervention, a reduction in these compensatory strategies was observed, along with improved trunk mobility and greater dissociation between the shoulder and pelvic girdles. Improvements in gait rhythm were also noted, contributing to a more automated and fluent walking pattern.

In addition to qualitative changes, quantitative gait parameters demonstrated functionally relevant improvements, as shown in Table 1. Gait speed increased, as demonstrated by the 10MWT result, surpassing the Minimal Clinically Important Difference (MCID) [8], enhancing day-to-day functional capacity and walking efficiency. Effort tolerance improved, as evidenced by the 6MWT results, reflecting greater functional endurance during daily activities. This enhancement exceeded the MCID [9], indicating a clinically meaningful gain in walking capacity. Furthermore, the perceived exertion during the test also decreased, suggesting an increased tolerance to physical effort. Dynamic balance also improved, particularly during gait as showed in TUG results, contributing to greater safety and a reduced risk of falls. A significant improvement in overall functional balance was also observed with the BBS score, which reflects not only improved gait stability but also enhanced performance in other balance-related activities. No episodes of excessive fatigue or adverse events were reported during the RAGT sessions.

4. Discussion

While robotic exoskeletons are primarily standardised to improve gait parameters [2], this case illustrates their potential to address broader motor goals related to overall gait pattern quality—including enhanced sensorimotor integration of the LLs, more effective weight transfer, and reduced reliance on compensatory strategies, as observed in the patient's gait. The patient's increased effort tolerance, along with improvements in gait velocity and dynamic balance (Table 1), further support this broader therapeutic value.

In addition to the qualitative observations, quantitative outcome measures also demonstrated significant progress. Gait speed increased, dynamic and functional balance improved, and effort tolerance rose across sessions. Importantly, some of the gains observed in walking assessments exceeded the MCID thresholds, reinforcing the clinical relevance of the intervention. The patient's BBS score improved, suggesting enhanced postural control, even though orthotic dependency and absence of movement in the left LL limited maximum scoring potential. Although the final BBS score did not reach the 40-point threshold associated with reduced fall risk, it still reflected meaningful improvements in balance and functional performance [9]. Furthermore, the interpretation should be contextualised: most BBS items are performed in an upright position, and the patient required both a KAFO and elbow crutches to maintain orthostasis due to the absence of active movement in the left LL. This limitation inherently restricted the scoring potential on the scale.

Despite the positive outcomes, certain limitations must be acknowledged. The effective duration of RAGT per session was shorter than current recommendations, which may have limited neuroplastic adaptation. Furthermore, although no adverse events or excessive fatigue were observed, the high cost and limited availability of exoskeleton devices remain significant barriers to widespread clinical implementation [4].

The integration of RAGT with an exoskeleton into a multidisciplinary paediatric rehabilitation programme proved to be a feasible and promising adjunct in the functional recovery of an adolescent with incomplete SCI due to idiopathic TM. In addition to improving spatiotemporal gait parameters, the intervention promoted more symmetrical weight distribution, reduced compensatory strategies, and enhanced gait balance, speed, and effort tolerance—key components for safe and efficient ambulation. These outcomes support the role of robotic technologies as valuable complements to conventional rehabilitation, particularly in paediatric populations where neuroplastic potential is high and long-term functional outcomes are critical. However, these findings are limited by the single-subject design. Kinematic analysis is also recommended to enhance the reliability of gait assessment beyond clinical observation. Further studies with larger cohorts and extended follow-up are warranted to confirm these preliminary results and to better understand the long-term effects of RAGT on neuroplasticity and autonomy.

5. Conclusions

This case supports the feasibility and therapeutic potential of integrating RAGT into paediatric neurorehabilitation. Clinically meaningful gains were observed in gait symmetry, weight transfer, and functional mobility. Despite limited training time and the single-case design, findings suggest exoskeletons may support broader motor goals beyond gait parameters. Further research is needed to explore long-term effects in promoting neuroplasticity and autonomy.

Author Contributions: Conceptualization, M.A.N.; methodology, M.A.N., A.L. and G.D.; formal analysis, M.A.N.; investigation, M.A.N., A.L., G.D., S.W., T.T., L.J., C.E.J. and I.B.; data curation, M.A.N., A.L. and G.D.; writing—original draft preparation, M.A.N.; writing—review and editing, M.A.N., A.L., G.D., S.W., T.T., L.J., C.E.J. and I.B.; visualisation, M.A.N. All authors have read and agreed to the published version of the manuscript.

Funding: This research received no external funding.

Informed Consent Statement: Informed consent was obtained from all subjects involved in the study.

Data Availability Statement: The data supporting the findings of this study are available from the corresponding author on reasonable request.

Acknowledgments: The authors are grateful to the patient and the family for their collaboration and consent in sharing this clinical case, which made this study possible.

Conflicts of Interest: The authors declare no conflicts of interest.

References

1. Celik, H.; Aksoy, E.; Oztoprak, U.; Ceylan, N.; Aksoy, A.; Yazici, M.U.; Azapagasi, E.; Eksioglu, A.S.; Yücel, H.; Senel, S.; et al. Longitudinally Extensive Transverse Myelitis in Childhood: Clinical Features, Treatment Approaches, and Long-Term Neurological Outcomes. *Clin. Neurol. Neurosurg.* **2021**, *207*, 106764. [CrossRef] [PubMed]
2. Nistor-Cseppento, C.D.; Gherle, A.; Negrut, N.; Bungau, S.G.; Sabau, A.M.; Radu, A.F.; Bungau, A.F.; Tit, D.M.; Uivaraseanu, B.; Ghitea, T.C.; et al. The Outcomes of Robotic Rehabilitation Assisted Devices Following Spinal Cord Injury and the Prevention of Secondary Associated Complications. *Medicina* **2022**, *58*, 1447. [CrossRef] [PubMed]
3. Zhang, Y.; Hui, Z.; Qi, W.; Zhang, J.; Wang, M.; Zhu, D. Clinical Study on the Safety and Feasibility of AiWalker-K for Lower Limbs Exercise Rehabilitation in Children with Cerebral Palsy. *PLoS ONE* **2024**, *19*, e0303517. [CrossRef] [PubMed]
4. Patathong, T.; Klaewkasikum, K.; Woratanarat, P.; Rattanasiri, S.; Anothaisintawee, T.; Woratanarat, T.; Thakkinstian, A. The Efficacy of Gait Rehabilitations for the Treatment of Incomplete Spinal Cord Injury: A Systematic Review and Network Meta-Analysis. *J. Orthop. Surg. Res.* **2023**, *18*, 60. [CrossRef] [PubMed]
5. Lefmann, S.; Russo, R.; Hillier, S. The Effectiveness of Robotic-Assisted Gait Training for Paediatric Gait Disorders: Systematic Review. *J. Neuroeng. Rehabil.* **2017**, *14*, 1. [CrossRef] [PubMed]
6. Liu, S.; Chen, F.; Yin, J.; Wang, G.; Yang, L. Comparative Efficacy of Robotic Exoskeleton and Conventional Gait Training in Patients with Spinal Cord Injury: A Meta-Analysis of Randomized Controlled Trials. *J. Neuroeng. Rehabil.* **2025**, *22*, 121. [CrossRef] [PubMed]
7. Glinsky, J.V.; Harvey, L.A.; Australian and New Zealand Physiotherapy Clinical Practice Guidelines Consortium. Australian and New Zealand Clinical Practice Guideline for the Physiotherapy Management of People with Spinal Cord Injury. Version 1.2. 2022. Available online: https://www.sciptguide.com (accessed on 25 June 2025).
8. Musselman, K.E.; Fouad, K.; Misiaszek, J.E.; Yang, J.F. Training of Walking Skills Overground and on the Treadmill: Case Series on Individuals with Incomplete Spinal Cord Injury. *Phys. Ther.* **2009**, *89*, 601–611. [CrossRef] [PubMed]
9. Forrest, G.F.; Hutchinson, K.; Lorenz, D.J.; Buehner, J.J.; Vanhiel, L.R.; Sisto, S.A.; Basso, D.M. Are the 10 Meter and 6 Minute Walk Tests Redundant in Patients with Spinal Cord Injury? *PLoS ONE* **2014**, *9*, e94108. [CrossRef] [PubMed]

medical sciences forum

MDPI

Proceeding Paper

Compensatory Muscle Activity Inhibition with Kinesiotape Application to the Unaffected Hemiface in a Person with Peripheral Facial Palsy: Two Case Reports †

Ana Cristina Sequeira [1,2,*], Cláudia Maria Costa [3], Wanda Neves [2], Sofia Pinto [1,2], Maria do Céu Nunes [2], António Ramos [2], Angela Maria Pereira [1,2,4] and Susana Almeida [2]

1 Physiotherapy Department, Egas Moniz School of Health & Science, Monte da Caparica, 2829-511 Almada, Portugal; sofiapinto@egasmoniz.edu.pt (S.P.); apereira@egasmoniz.edu.pt (A.M.P.)
2 Hospital Garcia de Orta, Unidade Local de Saúde Almada Seixal, 2805-267 Almada, Portugal; wanda.neves@ulsas.min-saude.pt (W.N.); maria.ceu.nunes@ulsas.min-saude.pt (M.d.C.N.); antonio.manuel.ramos@ulsas.min-saude.pt (A.R.); susana.farinha@ulsas.min-saude.pt (S.A.)
3 Physiotherapy Department, Escola Superior de Saúde Atlântica, 2730-036 Barcarena, Portugal; ccosta@uatlantica.pt
4 Egas Moniz Center for Interdisciplinary Research (CiiEM) Monte da Caparica, 2829-511 Almada, Portugal
* Correspondence: asequeira@egasmoniz.edu.pt
† Presented at the 7th CiiEM International Congress 2025—Empowering One Health to Reduce Social Vulnerabilities, Caparica, Portugal, 2–4 July 2025.

Abstract: Facial palsy (FP) is a nerve disorder causing unilateral facial muscle paralysis, impacting facial symmetry and non-verbal communication. This case study describes two idiopathic FP patients treated with physiotherapy and inhibitory kinesiotape (KT) applied to the unaffected side to reduce muscle hyperactivity. The intervention aimed to improve facial symmetry and psychological well-being. Both patients showed improvements in the Sunnybrook Facial Palsy Scale and the Hospital Anxiety and Depression Scale. Despite these promising outcomes, the small sample size limits our conclusions. Further controlled studies with larger samples are needed to confirm KT's effectiveness and clarify its role in FP rehabilitation.

Keywords: kinesiotape; facial palsy; peripheral facial paralysis; physiotherapy

1. Introduction

Facial palsy (FP) is a common neurological condition characterized by sudden unilateral facial paralysis due to facial nerve (VII) dysfunction. While FP has multiple potential causes—such as infections, trauma, neoplasms, and autoimmune disorders—the majority of cases are idiopathic, with Bell's palsy being the most frequent. Although often self-limiting, the sudden onset and uncertain course of FP can be distressing [1].

In addition to motor deficits, FP often leads to facial asymmetry, eye closure difficulties, and impaired oral function, impacting daily life. These limitations can result in significant psychosocial distress [2]. Although most cases recover within 3 to 4 weeks, delayed improvement during this period is associated with a higher risk of long-term impairment, underscoring the importance of early and effective rehabilitation [1–3].

Physiotherapy remains the primary approach in FP management, focusing on education, neuromuscular re-education, mirror therapy, proprioceptive training, and biofeedback-based techniques to facilitate neuromuscular control, prevent synkinesis, and promote facial symmetry. Recently, interest has grown in adjunct therapies to enhance these effects [3–6]. One such modality is kinesiotaping (KT), a non-invasive, elastic therapeutic taping method widely used in musculoskeletal and neurological rehabilitation [7,8].

KT is thought to act by modulating muscle tone, improving circulation, stimulating cutaneous mechanoreceptors, and enhancing the sensory and proprioceptive inputs. In FP, it is typically applied to the affected side to support weak muscles and promote neuromuscular activation [7,8]. However, KT may also be beneficial when applied to the unaffected side to inhibit compensatory overactivity [7]. Such excessive activation may disturb the interhemispheric balance, reinforce maladaptive patterns, and impede recovery by hindering proper activation of the affected side [1]. By modulating the sensory input and proprioceptive feedback, inhibitory KT may help regulate muscle tone and promote more symmetrical neuromuscular control. Despite its potential, the use of inhibitory KT on the unaffected side remains unexplored. Its rationale is grounded in the previously discussed motor control principles, emphasizing bilateral facial muscle interdependence [1].

This case report describes the clinical progression of two idiopathic facial palsy patients who received standard physiotherapy combined with inhibitory KT on the unaffected side, highlighting changes in their facial function, symmetry, and psychosocial outcomes to provide a comprehensive view of rehabilitation.

2. Materials and Methods

2.1. Study Design

This case report followed a prospective observational design and was conducted in alignment with the CARE (CAse REport) guidelines to ensure the completeness and transparency of clinical case reporting [9].

2.2. Clinical Cases

Two adult patients diagnosed with idiopathic facial palsy were evaluated and treated at an outpatient neurorehabilitation clinic. Each patient participated in a structured physiotherapy program over a four-month period, attending sessions three times per week, with each lasting approximately 45 min.

Case 1 involved a 65-year-old retired, active female who presented with sudden-onset right-sided facial paralysis, reporting that she woke up unable to close her right eye and smile properly and experienced facial heaviness and tightness. Case 2 was a 48-year-old male IT engineer with acute right-sided idiopathic facial palsy, who reported difficulty closing his right eye, flattening of the nasolabial fold, and dribbling while drinking.

For both patients, there was no preceding trauma, infection, or identifiable cause. Their medical histories were unremarkable, and neurological examinations confirmed isolated peripheral facial nerve involvement, consistent with a diagnosis of idiopathic facial palsy (Bell's palsy). Both received corticosteroid therapy and underwent 54 (Case 1) and 52 (Case 2) physiotherapy sessions. MRIs were performed in both cases due to delayed recovery, with no abnormal findings.

2.3. Assessment and Intervention Description

The patients were assessed at two time points, at session 13 (introduction KT) and at the end of the intervention period, as their initial progress was limited. The functional motor outcomes were evaluated using the Sunnybrook Facial Grading System (SFGS), which provides a more nuanced and quantitative evaluation. It assesses three domains: the resting facial symmetry, the symmetry of voluntary movement across five standard facial expressions, and the presence and severity of synkinesis. The scores from each domain are combined to yield a composite score ranging from 0 (complete paralysis) to 100 (normal function), allowing for sensitive tracking of clinical progress over time [10].

To assess the emotional and psychological impact of facial palsy, the Hospital Anxiety and Depression Scale (HADS) was administered at session 13 and post-intervention. The HADS is a validated 14-item self-report questionnaire designed to detect symptoms of anxiety (HADS-A) and depression (HADS-D) in patients with physical health conditions. Each subscale consists of 7 items, scored from 0 to 3, with total scores ranging from 0 to 21 per domain. Scores of 8 or above on either subscale are considered indicative of clinically relevant levels of anxiety or depression. The HADS is widely used in rehabilitation settings due to its sensitivity and its exclusion of somatic symptoms that might overlap with those of physical illness [11].

In addition to these standardized tools, we used qualitative observations documented by the treating therapist throughout the intervention period. These included notes on facial muscle coordination, compensatory patterns, tolerance to kinesiotaping, and subjective impressions of improvement [5].

The rehabilitation protocol included neuromuscular facilitation exercises aimed at enhancing voluntary muscle activation, proprioceptive stimulation using manual and tactile inputs, and verbal biofeedback training to promote neuromuscular control and reduce synkinesis. The patients were also educated on facial muscle awareness, posture correction, and relaxation techniques and were prescribed individualized home exercise programs [4,5].

In addition to standard care, KT was introduced as an adjunct therapy—starting in the fifth week for Case 1 and the third week for Case 2—following clinical reassessment due to delayed recovery. Using a low-tension inhibitory technique, with a stretch of 0 to 10%, administered from the muscle's insertion to its origin, elastic therapeutic tape was applied to the unaffected hemiface. The KT application was based on the criterion of targeting the hyperactive muscles identified during each session, which varied daily based on the physiotherapist's clinical assessment. These typically included the *frontalis, zygomaticus major and minor, and orbicularis oris muscles.* The purpose of KT application was to reduce the contralateral muscle hyperactivity on the unaffected side, aiming to promote functional symmetry by minimizing compensatory movements. Taping was performed every two days and maintained between sessions, with the patients instructed to keep the tape in place continuously unless irritation occurred. Their skin integrity and comfort were monitored.

2.4. Ethical Considerations

This study was conducted in accordance with the principles of the Declaration of Helsinki. Both participants provided written informed consent for participation and publication of anonymized data.

3. Results

Both participants demonstrated notable improvements in their facial muscle strength, dynamic symmetry, and psychosocial well-being over the course of the intervention. Improvements were observed both at rest and during voluntary facial movements, as measured by the SFGS and the HADS, as Figure 1 demonstrates.

Participant 1 showed a significant improvement in their SBFPS score, which increased from 25 to 88, indicating better voluntary movement, resting tone, and reduced synkinesis (see Figure 1a). Their HADS score decreased from 13 to 10, suggesting a mild reduction in anxiety and depression symptoms. Participant 2 exhibited a similar pattern, with their SBFPS score rising from 25 to 96, approaching full functional recovery, and a HADS score reduction from 9 to 3, reflecting a substantial decrease in psychological distress (see Figure 1b). Both participants also reported full functional recovery, with improved facial control, less social self-consciousness, and greater ease in their daily interactions. These reports were consistent with the physiotherapist's observations of enhanced neuromuscular coordination, reduced compensatory activity, and improved facial symmetry. No adverse effects were observed, and both patients completed the treatment protocol as planned.

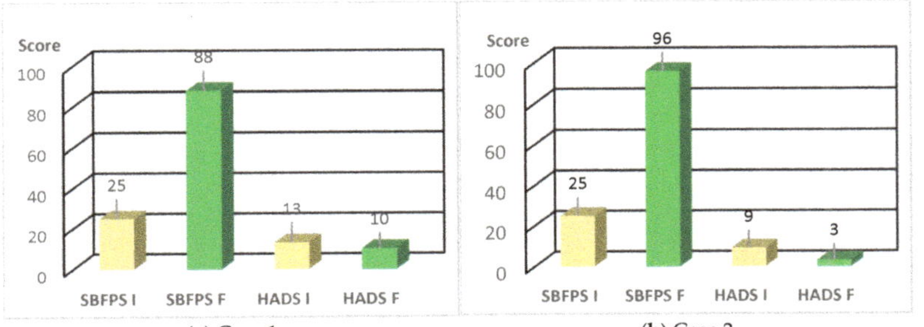

(**a**) Case 1 (**b**) Case 2

Figure 1. (**a**) Sunnybrook Facial Grading System (SBFPS) score and Hospital Anxiety and Depression Scale (HADS) score for Case 1 at the beginning of the KT application (I) and at the end (F); (**b**) SBFPS score and HADS score for Case 2 at the beginning of the application (I) and at the end (F).

4. Discussion

This case study provides preliminary evidence supporting the use of inhibitory KT as a complementary therapy in the rehabilitation of idiopathic FP. Both participants demonstrated improvements in their facial motor function and psychosocial well-being, with enhanced muscle strength, facial symmetry, and a reduction in psychological distress. These findings align with the current literature, which emphasizes the benefits of combining standard physiotherapy with adjunct therapies like KT [7].

The psychosocial outcomes were notably improved, with both participants reporting reduced anxiety and depression as measured by the HADS. This aligns with research suggesting that FP can cause significant psychological distress due to an altered facial appearance and difficulty in social interactions [2]. The reduction in the HADS scores reflects the positive emotional impact of improved facial symmetry and voluntary control, supporting the notion that rehabilitation of facial function contributes to better psychological well-being.

The innovative aspect of this case study was the inclusion of inhibitory KT on the unaffected hemiface to address compensatory hyperactivity—a factor that often complicates rehabilitation and hinders the long-term facial balance, particularly in cases of delayed recovery [1]. While KT is commonly used to facilitate muscle activity on the affected side [7], this approach aimed to modulate excessive activity on the unaffected side to promote more balanced muscle engagement between both hemifaces and prevent complications such as facial asymmetry and synkinesis development. Both participants showed a reduction in compensatory movements, which likely contributed to the overall improvement in their facial symmetry.

While our results are promising, several limitations must be acknowledged. First, this study employed a single-case design with a small sample size of only two participants. The absence of a control group limits our ability to attribute the observed improvements solely to the KT intervention. Future research should include larger sample sizes and randomized controlled trials to further evaluate the efficacy of KT in the rehabilitation of FP. Additionally, while both participants reported subjective improvements in their function and emotional well-being, more comprehensive psychosocial assessments, including qualitative interviews, would provide deeper insights into the emotional impact of facial rehabilitation.

5. Conclusions

These case reports highlight the potential benefits of adding inhibitory KT to standard physiotherapy for the treatment of idiopathic facial palsy, showing improvements in facial symmetry and psychological well-being. This novel approach warrants further investigation through randomized controlled trials to confirm its efficacy, determine the optimal application parameters, and establish clinical guidelines for its use in facial rehabilitation.

Author Contributions: Conceptualization, A.C.S. and C.M.C.; methodology, A.C.S.; formal analysis, A.C.S. and C.M.C.; investigation, A.C.S., S.P. and C.M.C.; resources, A.C.S., A.M.P., A.R. and S.A.; writing—original draft preparation, A.C.S. and C.M.C.; writing—review and editing, A.C.S., M.d.C.N., W.N. and C.M.C. All authors have read and agreed to the published version of the manuscript.

Funding: This research received no external funding.

Institutional Review Board Statement: This study was conducted in accordance with the Declaration of Helsinki.

Informed Consent Statement: Informed consent was obtained from all the subjects involved in the study.

Data Availability Statement: The data is unavailable due to privacy or ethical restrictions.

Acknowledgments: We would like to acknowledge the patients who allowed the use of their data for research purposes.

Conflicts of Interest: The authors declare no conflicts of interest.

References

1. Walker, N.R.; Mistry, R.K.; Mazzoni, T. Facial Nerve Palsy. In *StatPearls*; StatPearls Publishing: Treasure Island, FL, USA, 2025.
2. Hotton, M.; Huggons, E.; Hamlet, C.; Shore, D.; Johnson, D.; Norris, J.H.; Kilcoyne, S.; Dalton, L. The psychosocial impact of facial palsy: A systematic review. *Br. J. Health Psychol.* **2020**, *25*, 695–727. [CrossRef] [PubMed]
3. Nakano, H.; Fujiwara, T.; Tsujimoto, Y.; Morishima, N.; Kasahara, T.; Ameya, M.; Tachibana, K.; Sanada, S.; Toufukuji, S.; Hato, N. Physical therapy for peripheral facial palsy: A systematic review and meta-analysis. *Auris Nasus Larynx* **2024**, *51*, 154–160. [CrossRef] [PubMed]
4. Khan, A.J.; Szczepura, A.; Palmer, S.; Bark, C.; Neville, C.; Thomson, D.; Martin, H.; Nduka, C. Physical therapy for facial nerve paralysis (Bell's palsy): An updated and extended systematic review of the evidence for facial exercise therapy. *Clin. Rehabil.* **2022**, *36*, 1424–1449. [CrossRef] [PubMed]
5. Robinson, M.W.; Baiungo, J. Facial Rehabilitation: Evaluation and Treatment Strategies for the Patient with Facial Palsy. *Otolaryngol. Clin. N. Am.* **2018**, *51*, 1151–1167. [CrossRef] [PubMed]
6. Vaughan, A.; Gardner, D.; Miles, A.; Copley, A.; Wenke, R.; Coulson, S. A Systematic Review of Physical Rehabilitation of Facial Palsy. *Front. Neurol.* **2020**, *11*, 222. [CrossRef] [PubMed]
7. Di Stadio, A.; Gambacorta, V.; Ralli, M.; Pagliari, J.; Longari, F.; Greco, A.; Ricci, G. Facial taping as biofeedback to improve the outcomes of physical rehab in Bell's palsy: Preliminary results of a randomized case-control study. *Eur. Arch. Otorhinolaryngol.* **2021**, *278*, 1693–1698. [CrossRef] [PubMed]
8. Sun, Z.H.; Tian, Y.P.; Tan, Y.F.; Tao, D.; Li, W.B.; Ding, J.L.; Ai, S.C. Effectiveness of Kinesio taping on peripheral facial paralysis: A protocol for systematic review and meta-analysis. *Medicine* **2020**, *99*, e23090. [CrossRef] [PubMed]
9. Riley, D.S.; Barber, M.S.; Kienle, G.S.; Aronson, J.K.; von Schoen-Angerer, T.; Tugwell, P.; Kiene, H.; Helfand, M.; Altman, D.G.; Sox, H.; et al. CARE guidelines for case reports: Explanation and elaboration document. *J. Clin. Epidemiol.* **2017**, *89*, 218–235. [CrossRef] [PubMed]
10. Neely, J.G.; Cherian, N.G.; Dickerson, C.B.; Nedzelski, J.M. Sunnybrook facial grading system: Reliability and criteria for grading. *Laryngoscope* **2010**, *120*, 1038–1045. [CrossRef] [PubMed]
11. Beekman, E.; Verhagen, A. Clinimetrics: Hospital Anxiety and Depression Scale. *J. Physiother.* **2018**, *64*, 198. [CrossRef] [PubMed]

medical sciences forum

MDPI

Proceeding Paper

Satisfaction with Physiotherapy Care for Individuals with Cystic Fibrosis Across Face-to-Face, Online, and Blended Rehabilitation Settings †

Sofia O. Vieira [1,2,3,*], Ana Paula Martins [1,4], Ângela Pereira [1,4,5], Virgínia Marques [6], Inês Gano [2], Filipa Moita de Deus [1,7,8], Margarida Sousa [9] and Sónia Vicente [1,5]

1 Physiotherapy Department, Egas Moniz School of Health & Science, Caparica, 2829-511 Almada, Portugal; aplt@gmail.com (A.P.M.); apereira@egasmoniz.edu.pt (Â.P.); filipammd@gmail.com (F.M.d.D.); svicente@egasmoniz.edu.pt (S.V.)

2 Associação Nacional de Fibrose Quística, 1700-344 Alvalade, Portugal; ines.gano@gmail.com

3 Hospital de Santa Maria, Unidade Local de Saúde Santa Maria, 1649-028 Lisboa, Portugal

4 Hospital Garcia da Orta, Unidade Local de Saúde Almada-Seixal, 2805-267 Almada, Portugal

5 Egas Moniz Center for Interdisciplinary Research (CiiEM), Caparica, 2829-511 Almada, Portugal

6 Mirafisio, 1495-171 Algés, Portugal; virginia.marques.ft@gmail.com

7 Maternidade Alfredo da Costa, Unidade Local de Saúde São José, 1050-078 Lisboa, Portugal

8 Escola Superior de Tecnologia da Saúde de Lisboa, Instituto Politécnico de Lisboa, 1990-096 Lisboa, Portugal

9 Business School, Instituto Superior de Ciências do Trabalho e da Empresa-Instituto Universitário de Lisboa, 1649-026 Lisboa, Portugal; margaridafs2000@gmail.com

* Correspondence: scvieira@egasmoniz.edu.pt

† Presented at the 7th CiiEM International Congress 2025—Empowering One Health to Reduce Social Vulnerabilities, Caparica, Portugal, 2–4 July 2025.

Abstract: This study assessed satisfaction with physiotherapy care for individuals with cystic fibrosis across face-to-face, online, and blended formats at the National Association for Cystic Fibrosis. Forty participants, including patients and legal representatives, reported high satisfaction overall. Key strengths included respectful communication, involvement in decision-making, scheduling flexibility, and therapist support. Face-to-face care received the highest ratings, though privacy, understanding, and engagement were consistently strong across all modalities. The results highlight the importance of patient-centred approaches and suggest that high-quality care can be delivered effectively across different treatment formats, reinforcing satisfaction as a key indicator of healthcare quality and effectiveness.

Keywords: cystic fibrosis; physiotherapy; satisfaction; treatment modalities

1. Introduction

Patient satisfaction is a key indicator of healthcare quality, influenced by emotional, psychological, and personal factors, and plays a crucial role in assessing the potential and effectiveness of treatment [1–3]. Cystic fibrosis (CF) is an autosomal rare recessive disorder caused by mutations in the CF transmembrane conductance regulator gene, conventionally classified into six classes (I-VI) based on the resulting defect in protein synthesis or function [4]. This chronic, life-limiting disease requires multidisciplinary care in which physiotherapy plays a crucial role in maintaining lung function and slowing disease progression [5,6]. Care must be adaptable to each patient's evolving needs (i.e., health status and personal circumstances), especially for children and their families [7]. Traditionally, face-to-face programmes have represented the standard approach to CF management [8]. This setting offers hands-on care, real-time adjustments, access to specialised equipment,

 https://doi.org/10.3390/msf2025037013

multidisciplinary support between different health professionals, as well as immediate referral for hospital admission [7–9]. However, the COVID-19 pandemic prompted a rapid shift toward telemedicine, including online physiotherapy via video conferencing [8]. These online and hybrid modalities have improved accessibility—particularly for patients in rural and remote areas—by reducing travel time and associated costs [9]. In addition to this, remote exercise-based interventions offer flexibility, mitigate patient disinterest and lack of motivation [10,11], and minimise the risk of respiratory pathogen transmission, a critical concern for individuals with CF [8].

In Portugal, the National Association of Cystic Fibrosis (ANFQ) has supported individuals with CF since 1996 [12]. Since 2017, in collaboration with the Santa Maria Local Health Unit, ANFQ has offered free physiotherapy for children aged 6 months to 18 years in face-to-face, online, and blended formats. The selection of the most appropriate format depends on each child's individual needs, clinical condition, and geographical location. The objective of this study was to assess the perceived satisfaction of individuals with CF (aged 16 and older) and the legal representatives of younger patients (aged 15 and under) regarding the physiotherapy services at ANFQ across three treatment settings.

2. Materials and Methods

2.1. Study Design, Data Collection, and Participants

This cross-sectional observational study involved individuals with CF or their legal representatives regarding physiotherapy care from ANFQ. The total population of ANFQ was included in this study. All 41 eligible individuals were contacted by phone, with participation being voluntary, anonymous, and based on written informed consent. Inclusion required current use of ANFQ physiotherapy services; those without consent, with language barriers, or experiencing symptom exacerbation were excluded. Ethical approval was obtained from the Egas Moniz Ethics Committee. Data were collected online via Google Forms in May 2025 using the 43-item Patient Feedback Questionnaire (PFQ), previously validated for use in Portugal [13,14].

2.2. Statistical Analysis

Descriptive statistics (mean and standard deviation) were used to summarise satisfaction variables, while nominal and ordinal data were reported as percentages. To compare the data from the three rehabilitation settings, a Kruskal–Wallis test was conducted on Likert-scale items, as data did not follow a normal distribution. Statistical significance was set at $p < 0.05$. All tests were performed using Jamovi 2.6.44.

3. Results and Discussion

3.1. Participants Characterisation

The sample consisted of 40 participants, including 5 individuals with CF and 35 legal representatives. The mean age of individuals with CF was 19.2 years, while the legal representatives—responsible for children with CF—had a mean age of 41.91 years. Most respondents were female (n = 34). The sample was homogeneous in relation to the genotype, including class II and IV mutations, with the majority being class II, which is reflected in similar clinical manifestations. Treatment modalities included online (n = 14), face-to-face (n = 13), and blended (n = 13) rehabilitation. Each physical therapy session lasted 60 min. Participants in the blended and online modalities predominantly had treatment durations of over 4 years (n = 8 and n = 6, respectively), while the face-to-face group showed a more balanced distribution across all duration categories. Biweekly sessions were the most frequent across all modalities (face-to-face (n = 7), online (n = 9), and blended (n = 11)), followed by weekly sessions. Monthly and occasional sessions were reported only in the face-to-face and online groups.

3.2. Factors: Access to Care; Interpersonal Relationships; Active Participation

Most participants (n = 35) began physiotherapy within a month of their medical consultation, and 90.0% reported being able to choose their physiotherapy session schedules at ANFQ. This flexibility is essential for aligning physiotherapy with daily family routines, especially in paediatric care, and reflects strong support from physiotherapists toward patient and family needs [6]. All (n = 40) reported highly positive interactions with their physiotherapists, noting respectful communication, empathy, and attentiveness. Respondents unanimously confirmed being addressed by their preferred name, having their concerns and opinions listened to, and being treated with courtesy and sensitivity. In total, 97.5% rejected any discomfort or roughness in their care and confirmed feeling encouraged to express their preferences regarding treatment. Additionally, 95.0% reported full privacy and a clear understanding of the language used. These findings align with the World Confederation for Physiotherapy guidelines promoting holistic patient well-being [15]. Participants reported a high level of involvement in their physiotherapy care, with ample opportunities to ask questions, share opinions, and engage in treatment decisions. In total, 97.5% were informed of treatment benefits and risks, while a majority received multiple treatment options (73.7%) and were made aware of their right to refuse treatment (71.8%). Communication remained effective throughout: all participants understood treatment goals, most received feedback on progress (85.0%) and assessment results (97.5%) and were given clear instructions for home exercises (92.5%) and equipment use (94.8%). Nearly all also confirmed they were not asked to perform any unauthorised activities (97.5%). These results underscore a strong patient-centred approach, with clear and detailed communication fostering greater satisfaction [5]—consistent with findings from Jahan et al. on the role of effective communication in enhancing patient experience [16].

3.3. Satisfaction Level

This study revealed consistently high satisfaction with ANFQ's physiotherapy services and similar levels among the three groups. Legal representatives reported slightly higher scores (4.94 ± 0.23) than individuals with CF (4.80 ± 0.40). Most participants felt their expectations were met (legal representatives: 4.71 ± 0.85; CF patients: 4.80 ± 0.40) and strongly disagreed with the idea that physiotherapy was a waste of time (legal representatives: 4.91 ± 0.50; CF patients: 4.40 ± 1.20). These findings suggest a proactive and motivated attitude, likely contributing to greater involvement in treatment plans and, consequently, greater satisfaction. Additionally, meeting patient expectations plays a crucial role in satisfaction, with user-reported satisfaction significantly increasing when expectations are fulfilled [17]. Among modalities, 3-4 years of face-to-face care weekly achieved the highest satisfaction level (5.00 ± 0.00), followed by blended (4.92 ± 0.27) and online formats (4.86 ± 0.35).

Kruskal–Wallis did not show significant differences ($p > 0.05$) while comparing all Likert-scale items from the three rehabilitation settings. Despite this, a descriptive analysis of the items revealed three key findings. Regarding privacy, satisfaction levels were consistently high across all settings, with participants in the online group reporting the highest average scores, indicating that remote participation did not compromise their sense of privacy. Concerning communication, participants who had direct contact with the physiotherapist—either in face-to-face or blended settings—reported slightly higher average scores, suggesting that physical presence may enhance the perception of communication quality. Lastly, when it came to involvement in decision-making and the ability to express opinions during physiotherapy sessions, as well as being treated with courtesy and respect, there were no notable differences between the settings, indicating that patients felt equally engaged and heard regardless of how the sessions were delivered and reinforcing the consistency of interpersonal interactions across modalities. These findings align with the principles outlined by the World Confederation for Physical Therapy [15], particularly regarding ethical principles, patient-centred care, communication, and respect.

4. Conclusions

High levels of satisfaction with physiotherapy services at ANFQ were found, both among individuals with CF and their legal representatives, particularly in face-to-face settings. Although important, these findings may not be generalisable to all individuals with CF in Portugal. Moreover, as with most satisfaction voluntary surveys, there is a possibility of response bias, where more satisfied users may have been more inclined to participate. The absence of qualitative data also limits a deeper understanding of the reasons behind the satisfaction ratings. Nonetheless, this study highlights the importance of systematically assessing satisfaction to better understand patient experiences across different treatment modalities, contributing to more responsive, equitable, and patient-centred physiotherapy care.

Author Contributions: Conceptualization, S.O.V. and S.V.; formal analysis, S.O.V., A.P.M., and Â.P.; investigation, S.O.V.; writing—original draft preparation, S.O.V.; writing—review and editing, Â.P., V.M., I.G., F.M.d.D., M.S., and S.V.; supervision, S.V. All authors have read and agreed to the published version of the manuscript.

Funding: This research received no external funding.

Institutional Review Board Statement: The study was conducted in accordance with the Declaration of Helsinki and approved by the Egas Moniz Ethics Committee (Process No. 1593 of 30/04/2025).

Informed Consent Statement: Informed consent was obtained from all subjects involved in the study.

Data Availability Statement: The data will be made available by the corresponding author upon request.

Acknowledgments: The authors acknowledge the ANFQ board and all patients or legal representatives for their collaboration in this study.

Conflicts of Interest: The authors declare no conflicts of interest.

References

1. Batbaatar, E.; Dorjdagva, J.; Luvsannyam, A.; Amenta, P. Conceptualisation of Patient Satisfaction: A Systematic Narrative Literature Review. *Perspect. Public Health* **2015**, *135*, 243–250. [CrossRef] [PubMed]
2. Vaitsman, J.; Andrade, G.R.B.d. Satisfação e Responsividade: Formas de Medir a Qualidade e a Humanização Da Assistência à Saúde. *Cien. Saude Colet.* **2005**, *10*, 599–613. [CrossRef]
3. Gutiérrez-Sánchez, D.; Cruzado, D.; Cuesta-Vargas, A. Instruments for Measuring Satisfaction with Physical Therapy Care: A Systematic Review. *Phys. Ther.* **2020**, *100*, 1690–1700. [CrossRef] [PubMed]
4. Elborn, J.S. Cystic Fibrosis. *Lancet* **2016**, *388*, 2519–2531. [CrossRef] [PubMed]
5. Byrne, N.M.; Hardy, L. Community Physiotherapy for Children with Cystic Fibrosis: A Family Satisfaction Survey. *J. Cyst. Fibros.* **2005**, *4*, 123–127. [CrossRef] [PubMed]
6. Andrews, K.; Smith, M.; Cox, N.S. Physiotherapy: At What Cost? Parents Experience of Performing Chest Physiotherapy for Infants with Cystic Fibrosis. *J. Child Health Care* **2020**, *25*, 616–627. [CrossRef] [PubMed]
7. Doumit, M.; Pacey, V.; Jaffe, A.; Gray, K. Understanding the Acceptability of the Changing Model of Care in Cystic Fibrosis. *Respir. Med.* **2024**, *234*, 107847. [CrossRef] [PubMed]
8. Shanthikumar, S.; Ruseckaite, R.; Corda, J.; Mulrennan, S.; Ranganathan, S.; Douglas, T. Telehealth Use in Australian Cystic Fibrosis Centers:Clinician Experiences. *Pediatr. Pulmonol.* **2023**, *58*, 2906–2915. [CrossRef] [PubMed]
9. Wood, J.; Mulrennan, S.; Hill, K.; Cecins, N.; Morey, S.; Jenkins, S. Telehealth Clinics Increase Access to Care for Adults with Cystic Fibrosis Living in Rural and Remote Western Australia. *J. Telemed. Telecare* **2016**, *23*, 673–679. [CrossRef] [PubMed]

10. Poulsen, M.; Holland, A.E.; Button, B.; Jones, A.W. Preferences and Perspectives Regarding Telehealth Exercise Interventions for Adults with Cystic Fibrosis: A Qualitative Study. *Pediatr. Pulmonol.* **2024**, *59*, 1217–1226. [CrossRef] [PubMed]
11. Fainardi, V.; Capoferri, G.; Tornesello, M.; Pisi, G.; Esposito, S. Telemedicine and Its Application in Cystic Fibrosis. *J. Pers. Med.* **2023**, *13*, 1041. [CrossRef] [PubMed]
12. ANFQ—Associação Nacional de Fibrose Quística. Available online: http://www.anfq.pt/a-anfq/ (accessed on 2 June 2025).
13. Bettencourt, C.; Machado, I.M.; Fonseca, J.P.; Pascoalinho, J.; Avillez, M.; Murta, O.; Amado, S. *Instrumentos de Auditoria Aos Padrões de Prática*; Associação Portuguesa de Fisioterapeutas: Oeiras, Portugal, 2005.
14. Barros, M.G.M.; Lopes, A.M.F.; Pascoalinho, J. *Contributo Para Adaptação e Validação Para a Realidade Portuguesa Do Questionário de Audição Do Utente*; Monografia Final de Curso de Licenciatura Em Fisioterapia; Escola Superior de Saúde de Alcoitão: Alcoitão, Portugal, 2002; pp. 43–45.
15. WCPT. *Description of Physical Therapy: Policy Statement*; World Confederation for Physical Therapy: London, UK, 2019; pp. 1–8.
16. Jahan, A.M.; Rwaiha, A.E.; Gusaibat, S.R.; Al-Ahwal, N.A.; Al-Jafairi, Z.M.; Al-Rashidi, M.A. Patient Satisfaction with Physiotherapy Services in Libya: A Cross-Sectional Study. *J. Patient Exp.* **2021**, *8*, 1–7. [CrossRef] [PubMed]
17. Rossettini, G.; Latini, T.M.; Palese, A.; Jack, S.M.; Ristori, D.; Gonzatto, S.; Testa, M. Determinants of Patient Satisfaction in Outpatient Musculoskeletal Physiotherapy: A Systematic, Qualitative Meta-Summary, and Meta-Synthesis. *Disabil. Rehabil.* **2018**, *42*, 460–472. [CrossRef] [PubMed]

medical sciences forum

MDPI

Proceeding Paper

Compassion Fatigue in Portuguese Firefighters: Preliminary Results of the Compassion Fatigue Scale †

Lucas Sousa [1], Joana Antunes [1], Bruna Dias [1], Adriana Coelho [1], Karolina Costa [1], Andreia Conceição [1], Marina Carvalho [1,2,3,*], Carla Tomás [1] and Mária Viegas [1]

1 Department of Psychology and Physical Education, Instituto Superior Manuel Teixeira Gomes (ISMAT), 8500-590 Portimão, Portugal; lucasunisousa@gmail.com (L.S.); joana.demagalhaes.antunes@gmail.com (J.A.); brunaalexandradias2003@gmail.com (B.D.); adrianacscoelho@gmail.com (A.C.); karoollcostaa16@gmail.com (K.C.); p5817@ismat.pt (A.C.); p3190@ismat.pt (C.T.); p7448@ismat.pt (M.V.)
2 Psychiatry Service, Unidade Local de Saúde do Algarve (ULS Algarve), 8500-338 Portimão, Portugal
3 Instituto de Saúde Ambiental (ISAMB), 1649-026 Lisboa, Portugal
* Correspondence: marina.carvalho@ismat.pt
† Presented at the 7th CiiEM International Congress 2025—Empowering One Health to Reduce Social Vulnerabilities, Caparica, Portugal, 2–4 July 2025.

Abstract: The present study had the purpose of creating and studying the psychometric properties of the Compassion Fatigue Scale (CFS) in a sample of 286 firefighters, 69% of whom were males and 78% had previous exposure to a limit situation. All participants were assessed after their informed consent through a protocol composed of a sociodemographic data section, the CFS and the Professional Quality of Life scale (ProQOL). The CFS evidenced a two-dimensional structure, Compassion Fatigue and Compassion Satisfaction, with Cronbach's alphas superior to 0.90 and correlations in the expected direction with ProQOL. Females showed higher levels of compassion fatigue than males, demonstrating that CFS can be a reliable and valid self-report measure of compassion fatigue in firefighters.

Keywords: compassion fatigue; compassion satisfaction; firefighters; burnout; secondary traumatic stress

1. Introduction

Burnout and, specifically, compassion fatigue, a distinct form of burnout that can occur in persons regularly exposed to trauma and suffering (as is the case with hospital emergency and pre-emergency professionals), is an emergent health topic, due to its medium- and long-term impact on health. However, to the best of our knowledge, there is only one measure of compassion fatigue, directed to the general population.

Compassion fatigue is a specific form of burnout that can arise in individuals, professionals or even informal caregivers, resulting from systematic exposure to the suffering of others, which can lead to vicarious traumatization and cumulative burnout [1–3]. Thus, compassion fatigue is more likely to occur in health professionals and the pre-hospital emergency area, and in professionals in security, protection and social services, who are increasingly exposed to risks related to the social determinants of health throughout development. Literature reviews carried out in this area among health professionals have shown that the determinants of compassion fatigue include individual, organizational and ecosystem-related factors [4] and that, among the main consequences are its impact on the quality of care provided on personal and family life [4,5] and on mental health [5]. Firefighters are one of the professions constantly exposed to extreme situations that can lead to vicarious traumatization, as they are constantly called upon to intervene in situations of which they may have little or no knowledge and which require rapid and effective decision-making [6]. Studies carried out with firefighters highlight the negative impact on well-being caused by exposure to traumatic events and the greater likelihood of developing compassion fatigue [7]. On the other hand, compassion satisfaction, that is, the positive feeling of accomplishment and gratification that results from providing help to others and its impact on other people's lives, may constitute a protective factor that can buffer compassion fatigue [8].

However, despite the relevance of the topic, there are still few studies conducted with firefighters, highlighting the need to develop measures to assess this specific population. The measure probably most widely used in this context is the ProQOL [9], a self-report measure of professional quality of life which measures burnout, secondary traumatic stress (compassion fatigue) and compassion satisfaction. In Portugal, to our knowledge, there is only one measure adapted for this purpose in firefighters, the Compassion Fatigue-Short Scale [10], which, in the original, was constructed to assess compassion fatigue in social workers [11] but does not assess compassion satisfaction.

Thus, the main goal of the present study was to develop and study the preliminary psychometric qualities of a compassion fatigue self-report in firefighters. It was expected that the obtained dimensions would present adequate levels of reliability and validity.

2. Materials and Methods

2.1. Participants

Participants were included in this cross-sectional study if they were active firefighters over 18, working in any region of the country.

2.2. Measures

The ProQOL is a self-report measure of compassion fatigue, composed of 30 items which assess the frequency of each experience in the 30 days before the assessment in a 5-point Likert scale (1, Never; 5, Very Frequently) in three dimensions: compassion satisfaction (CS), burnout and secondary traumatic stress. The ProQOL presents adequate psychometric properties, with Cronbach's alphas superior to 0.71 [12]. The CFS was developed within the scope of the present study, and the results of its psychometric properties will be presented in the Results Section. The studied measure consisted of 28 items for which participants were asked to rate the frequency with which they usually experienced the described in each item, according to a 5-point Likert scale (1, Never; 5, Always).

2.3. Procedures

An initial set of items was developed and reviewed to reflect a comprehensive set of experiences across different categories of compassion fatigue. These items were first analyzed for their face and content validity. The research protocol, composed of an informed consent section, a sociodemographic section and both self-report measures, was then subjected to validation, and a pilot study was carried out with the main goal of clarifying potential language and response doubts and understanding the duration of the protocol administration. After small revisions and institutional board approval, the protocol was disseminated through different firefighters' corporations all over the country, with a request addressed to each commander to disseminate the study among the firefighters of their corporation. The protocol was available online between May and October 2024 and had an average filling time of 10 min.

2.4. Statistical Procedures

Face and content validity were assessed through interrater agreement. The internal structure of CFS was studied through exploratory factor analyses. Reliability was studied through Cronbach's alphas and intercorrelations, and concurrent validity was studied through Pearson's correlations. Comparisons between groups were studied through independent Student's *t* tests (assuming normality), and descriptive statistics were calculated for CFS norms. A confidence level of 95% was considered for each of the analyses.

3. Results

3.1. Sociodemographic Characteristics of the Participants

A convenience sample composed of 286 volunteer and professional firefighters from different corporations across the country was studied, which included 88 (31%) females and 198 (69%) males, aged between 18 and 63 years old ($M = 38.48$, $SD = 10.19$). Most of the participants reported working as firefighters for 8 to over 20 years (66.8%). Most of the participants spent at least 12 years in school (96%), and more than half of the participants were married or reported living with another person (53%). Also, 78% of the participants reported being already exposed to limit situations, and more than half of the participants reported working more than 35 h/week (53%).

3.2. Face and Content Validity of the Compassion Fatigue Scale

An initial pool of 35 items was developed and submitted to a panel of two non-experts and two experts to assess their facial and content validity, respectively. Based on the interrater agreement (IA) results, 7 of the 35 items were excluded due to ambiguity or because they did not represent the dimensions of compassion fatigue that were intended to be assessed (IA inferior to 49%), 17 of the items were included in the preliminary test version (IA superior to 75%), and 11 of the items were subjected to reformulation (IA between 50 and 74%). The final testing version was composed of 28 items.

3.3. Internal Structure of the Compassion Fatigue Scale

The internal structure of the 28 items of the CFS was studied through exploratory factor analyses with principal axis factorization and Varimax rotation. Based on principal components, the factorial solution was determined according to the following criteria: KMO and Bartlet's test (KMO = 0.91, χ^2 (35) = 4574.49, $p < 0.001$), eigenvalues superior to 1, explained variance superior to 50%, loadings superior to 0.40, ambiguity (difference superior to 0.30 when loading on more than one factor) and scree plot.

Only one item was excluded, and the results of a scree test pointed to a structure composed of two factors. A subsequent exploratory factor analysis was conducted with the 27 retained items. The first factor, Compassion Fatigue (CF), was composed of 17 items related to emotional, cognitive, physiological and social distress, and the second factor, Compassion Satisfaction (CS), was composed of 11 items related to positive feelings about the impact of work on other persons. Both factors explained about 48% of the total variance.

3.4. Reliability

Internal consistency values, Cronbach's alphas, were equal to 0.91 (CF) and 0.93 (CS). Inter-item correlations varied from 0.12 to 0.77, and item-total correlations were between 0.45 and 0.87. The intercorrelation between the two dimensions was equal to 0.18 ($p = 0.002$).

3.5. Concurrent Validity

Positive moderate correlations were found between CFS-CF with ProQOL Burnout ($r = 0.36$, $p < 0.001$) and Secondary Traumatic Stress ($r = 0.63$, $p < 0.001$). Positive moderate correlations were also found between CFS-CS with ProQOL-CS ($r = 0.61$, $p < 0.001$). A negative moderate correlation was obtained between CFS-CS and ProQOL Burnout ($r = -0.49$, $p = 0.001$). CFS-CF was independent of ProQOL-CS ($r = 0.007$, $p > 0.05$), and CFS-CS was independent of ProQOL Secondary Traumatic Stress ($r = -0.04$, $p > 0.05$).

3.6. Comparisons Between Groups

Comparisons between groups were carried out through t tests for independent samples. Significant sex differences were found for compassion fatigue, t (284) = 3.49, $p = 0.0005$. Female firefighters reported higher levels of compassion fatigue ($M = 46.9$, $SD = 10.3$) compared to male firefighters ($M = 42.9$, $SD = 5.3$). No significant sex differences were found for compassion satisfaction t (284) = 1.44, $p = 0.151$. Also, no significant group differences were found in compassion fatigue, t (284) = −0.29, $p = 0.77$, and compassion satisfaction, t (284) = −1.17, $p = 0.24$, when comparing firefighters who reported already being exposed to a limit situation with firefighters not exposed to a limit situation.

3.7. Norms

The resulting norms in the present sample are presented in Table 1.

Table 1. CFS norms.

	N	M	SD	Range	P^{25}	P^{50}	P^{75}	Sk	K
Compassion fatigue	286	43.69	10.57	17–82	36	43	50	0.50	0.74
Compassion satisfaction	286	41.99	10.00	10–50	39	44	47	−1.70	3.74

Note. Sk = Skewness; K = Kurtosis.

4. Discussion

The present study had the main goal of developing and studying the preliminary psychometric qualities of the CFS in firefighters. As expected, the obtained dimensions revealed adequate reliability and validity. The internal structure was adequate, and although there were some differences (compassion fatigue and burnout seem to be understood as different components on the same dimension), it seems to reflect the theoretical model [2,3] on which it was based. Correlations with the ProQOL and sex differences were also in the expected direction and according to the literature [10,13]. Despite the importance of the results, the present study has limitations, related to the sample (not random) and study nature (cross-sectional). Future studies are needed to replicate the invariance of the structure and assess its temporal stability. Although exploratory, the results are of most relevance for theory and professional practice. Interventions aimed at preventing compassion fatigue should promote self-care, the identification and recognition of its early manifestations and communication (horizontal and vertical) and support. Also, there is a need for systematic monitoring of these interventions to identify the mental health impact of CF and to provide targeted, timely and appropriate resources for its prevention.

5. Conclusions

The obtained results demonstrated that CFS can be a reliable and valid self-report measure of compassion fatigue in firefighters, and results highlight the relevance of the inclusion of sociodemographic variables in the interventions designed to prevent compassion fatigue in vulnerable populations.

Author Contributions: Conceptualization, L.S., J.A., B.D., K.C., M.C. and A.C. (Andreia Conceição); methodology, L.S., J.A., B.D., A.C. (Adriana Coelho), K.C., M.C. and A.C. (Andreia Conceição); validation, M.C. and A.C. (Andreia Conceição); formal analysis, M.C. and A.C. (Andreia Conceição); investigation, L.S., J.A., B.D., A.C. (Adriana Coelho), K.C., M.C. and A.C. (Andreia Conceição); resources, A.C. (Andreia Conceição), M.C., C.T. and M.V.; data curation, M.C. and A.C. (Andreia Conceição); writing—original draft preparation, M.C.; writing—review and editing, L.S., J.A., B.D., M.C., A.C. (Andreia Conceição), and M.V.; visualization, M.C.; supervision, M.C. and A.C. (Andreia Conceição); project administration, M.C. and A.C. (Andreia Conceição). All authors have read and agreed to the published version of the manuscript.

Funding: This research received no external funding.

Institutional Review Board Statement: The study was conducted in accordance with the Declaration of Helsinki and approved by the Institutional Review Board (11 March 2024, P2425-11).

Informed Consent Statement: Informed consent was obtained from all subjects.

Data Availability Statement: All data and materials are available upon request from Marina Carvalho, data bank manager, due to privacy and ethical reasons.

Conflicts of Interest: The authors declare no conflicts of interest.

References

1. Cocker, F.; Joss, N. Compassion Fatigue among Healthcare, Emergency and Community Service Workers: A Systematic Review. *Int. J. Environ. Res. Public Health* **2016**, *13*, 618. [CrossRef] [PubMed]
2. Figley, C.R. Compassion fatigue: Psychotherapists' chronic lack of self care. *J. Clin. Psychol.* **2002**, *58*, 1433–1441. [CrossRef] [PubMed]
3. Figley, C.R. Compassion fatigue as secondary traumatic stress disorder: An overview. In *Compassion Fatigue: Coping with Secondary Traumatic Stress Disorder in Those Who Treat the Traumatized*; Figley, C.R., Ed.; Brunner-Routledge: London, UK, 1995; pp. 1–20.
4. Garnett, A.; Hui, L.; Oleynikov, C.; Boamah, S. Compassion fatigue in healthcare providers: A scoping review. *BMC Health Serv. Res.* **2023**, *23*, 1336. [CrossRef] [PubMed]
5. Lluch, C.; Galiana, L.; Doménech, P.; Sansó, N. The Impact of the COVID-19 Pandemic on Burnout, Compassion Fatigue, and Compassion Satisfaction in Healthcare Personnel: A Systematic Review of the Literature Published during the First Year of the Pandemic. *Healthcare* **2022**, *10*, 364. [CrossRef] [PubMed]
6. García-Iglesias, J.J.; Bermejo-Ramírez, A.M.; Goniewicz, K.; Fernández-Carrasco, F.J.; Gómez-Salgado, C.; Camacho-Vega, J.C.; Gómez-Salgado, J. Predictive stressors for the burnout syndrome in firefighters. A systematic review. *Saf. Sci.* **2025**, *186*, 106831. [CrossRef]
7. Gonzalez, T.C.; Burnett, H.J.; Helm, H.; Edwards, L. An examination of resilience, compassion fatigue, burnout, and compassion satisfaction between men and women among trauma responders. *N. Am. J. Psych.* **2019**, *21*, 1–20.
8. McDonald, M.A.; Meckes, S.J.; Lancaster, C.L. Compassion for Oneself and Others Protects the Mental Health of First Responders. *Mindfulness* **2021**, *12*, 659–671. [CrossRef] [PubMed]
9. Stamm, B.H. *The Concise ProQOL Manual*; ProQOL.org: Pocatello, ID, USA, 2010.
10. Rodrigues, F.; Bártolo, A.; Sabino, D.; Santos, I.M.; Pereira, A.; Silva, C.F.; Boscarino, J.A.; Adams, R.E. Validation of the Compassion Fatigue Short Scale among Portuguese firefighters. *Anál. Psicol.* **2023**, *41*, 69–85. [CrossRef]
11. Adams, R.E.; Figley, C.R.; Boscarino, J.A. The Compassion Fatigue Scale: Its use with social workers following urban disaster. *Res. Soc. Work Pract.* **2008**, *18*, 238–250. [CrossRef] [PubMed]
12. Carvalho, P. Estudo da fadiga por compaixão nos cuidados paliativos em Portugal: Tradução e adaptação cultural da escala "Professional Quality of Life 5". Unpublished Master's Thesis, Universidade Católica Portuguesa, Porto, Portugal, 2011.
13. Burnett, H.J. Revisiting the Compassion Fatigue, Burnout, Compassion Satisfaction, and Resilience Connection Among CISM Responders. *SAGE Open J. Police Emerg. Resp.* **2017**, *7*, 1–10. [CrossRef]

medical sciences forum

MDPI

Proceeding Paper

Ventilatory Profile of Big Wave Surfers: An Exploratory Study †

Pedro Seixas [1,2], Ana Laura-Ricci-Vitor [1] and Lara Costa e Silva [1,*]

1 Escola Superior de Saúde Atlântica, Fábrica da Pólvora de Barcarena, 2730-036 Barcarena, Portugal; pseixas@uatlantica.pt (P.S.); aricci@uatlantica.pt (A.L.-R.-V.)
2 Surfing Medicine International, Van bylandtstraat 135, 2562 GB The Hague, The Netherlands
* Correspondence: laras@uatlantica.pt
† Presented at the 7th CiiEM International Congress 2025—Empowering One Health to Reduce Social Vulnerabilities, Caparica, Portugal, 2–4 July 2025.

Abstract: Big wave surfing, a high-risk sport involving rides on waves over 30 feet tall, exposes athletes to intense physical demands, particularly during wipeouts requiring extended breath-holding (apnea). Despite its growing popularity and professional status, the ventilatory profile of these elite athletes remains underexplored. This study is the first to examine the respiratory characteristics of Big Wave Surfers (BWS), focusing on lung function, respiratory muscle strength, and potential ventilatory adaptations or compromises. Findings suggest that BWS exhibit enhanced respiratory capacity, likely from apnea training and glossopharyngeal breathing, but also show signs of small airway obstruction, warranting further investigation and preventive health strategies.

Keywords: surfing; big waves; apnea; pulmonary function; respiratory muscles

1. Introduction

Big wave surfing is an extreme surfing discipline, defined by riding waves exceeding 30 feet (approximately 9 m) in height [1]. In big wave surfing, the physical demands escalate significantly, particularly during wipeouts, where athletes may be forced to hold their breath (apnea) for extended periods while subjected to strong underwater turbulence and pressure. To perform at an elite level, surfers must possess a combination of muscular endurance, upper-body strength, anaerobic power, and exceptional cardiorespiratory fitness [2]. Unlike most land-based athletes, surfers—especially in big wave surfing—are often submerged, exposed to cold water, and subjected to repeated apnea episodes. Therefore, it is plausible that their respiratory system adapts and presents superior lung capacities in ways similar to swimmers [3,4] or free divers [5,6]. Moreover, similarly to free-divers, before an apnea, Big Wave Surfers (BWS) also utilize Glossopharyngeal breathing (GPB) (or "frog breathing") as a strategy to pack more air into their lungs after a deep breath, in order to increase their total lung capacity between 0.5 and 3 L [7,8], and increase residual lung volume and intra-thoracic pressure [9]. However, the long-term consequences of this technique are not yet entirely clear, and some risks associated with its continued practice (e.g., barotrauma; pulmonary hypertension) have been reported [4].

This study aims to examine the respiratory adaptations associated with big wave surfing and whether the physical stressors inherent to the sport lead to functional or structural pulmonary changes.

2. Materials and Methods

This is a cross-sectional, exploratory epidemiological study. The sample was composed of 17 professional big wave surfing athletes (18–52 years old), selected through convenience sampling. Inclusion criteria required individuals to have competed in at least one official national or international BWS competition. Exclusion criteria included having a current infection, chest discomfort, a history of serious pulmonary disease or thoracic injury such as rib fractures, or any musculoskeletal or pulmonary injury in the six months prior to the study. To minimize potential fatigue-related bias, all data were collected before any physical activity or surf sessions. Participant characterization was achieved through a structured questionnaire that gathered demographic information and details about their surfing practice. Anthropometric variables included height and body mass, which were measured using calibrated portable equipment. Pulmonary function in a forced maneuver was evaluated using a portable spirometer (MIR SPIROLAB II, MIR slr, Rome, Italy) following the guideline recommendations [10]. Respiratory muscle strength was assessed by measuring maximal inspiratory pressure (MIP) and maximal expiratory pressure (MEP), using a MicroRPM (Vyaire Medical GmbH, Höchberg, Germany) pressure manometer. Participants were seated and used a nasal clip during testing. For MIP, subjects performed a slow and complete exhalation followed by a strong, rapid inhalation for at least 1.5 s. For MEP, after a maximal slow inhalation, they exhaled forcefully and quickly. Each of these measures was repeated 3 times with a minimum 1 min rest between trials, and tests were conducted in a temperature-controlled environment between 18° and 22 °C. For the statistical analysis the normality was assessed by the Kolmogorov–Smirnov test. Paired t-tests were applied to compare actual and predicted values for both spirometry and respiratory pressures. Multiple linear regression was used to identify significant correlations between variables such as age, years of surfing experience, and years of big wave surfing with pulmonary function measures. A significance level of $p < 0.05$ was adopted. All statistical analyses were performed using Microsoft Excel and IBM SPSS Statistics version 27.0.

3. Results

The 17 BWS athletes were male individuals (n = 14; 82.35%), with an average age of 33 ± 8.50 years. Their average surfing experience was 24.59 ± 7.53 years, and big wave surfing experience ranged from "less than 5 years" (n = 3; 17.64%), "6 to 7 years" (n = 4; 23.52%), to "more than 9 years" (n = 10; 58.82%). It is also evident that this sample is highly representative of the global elite, as all participants had competed in at least one big wave surfing competition, with 7 of them (41.17%) having participated more than seven times. Furthermore, the majority (n = 15; 82.35%) had already received BWS awards or award-nominations. Table 1 shows the average values of the ventilatory parameters of BWS, as well as the predicted values. For muscle strength, analyzed by MIP and MEP, it is possible to verify in Table 2 that all values, despite being higher in relation to the predicted values, do not present a statistically significant difference, except for MIP in male BWS. No other statistically significant relationships were found between lung function parameters and variables such as age or years of practice (surfing and/or big wave surfing).

Table 1. Spirometry ventilatory parameters of Big Wave Surfers—mean and predicted values.

Variables	Scores	Predicted Scores	Predicted Scores (%)	p
FVC (L)	6.28 ± 1.42	4.68 ± 0.69	134.29 ± 21.92	<0.001 **
FEV1 (L)	4.73 ± 0.85	3.92 ± 0.56	120.94 ± 15.63	<0.001 **
FEV1/FVC (%)	76.19 ± 6.17	81.51 ± 1.43	93.47 ± 7.34	<0.001 **
PEF (L/s)	10.54 ± 2.26	9.10 ± 1.17	115.71 ± 18.53	0.002 *
$FEF_{25–75\%}$ (L/s)	4.21 ± 0.77	4.55 ± 0.48	93.00 ± 16.95	0.044 *

Abbreviations: FVC: Forced Vital Capacity; FEV1: Forced Expiratory Volume in the first second; PEF: Peak Expiratory Flow; $FEF_{25–75\%}$: Average Forced Expiratory Flow; * $p < 0.05$; ** $p < 0.001$.

Table 2. Maximum respiratory pressures (MRP) of Big Wave Surfers.

Variables	Score	Predicted Score	p
MIP (cmH_2O)	138.35 ± 29.03	n.a.	n.a.
♂ (n = 14)	143.36 ± 25.72	106.85 ± 3.77	<0.001 *
♀ (n = 3)	114 ± 36.71	86.85 ± 2.88	0.178
MEP (cmH_2O)	143.88 ± 27.89	n.a.	n.a.
♂ (n = 14)	149.57 ± 23.69	147.38 ± 7.63	0.372
♀ (n = 3)	117.33 ± 35.92	101.18 ± 4.06	0.276

Abbreviations: MIP: maximum inspiratory pressure; MEP: maximum expiratory pressure; ♂: male; ♀: female; * $p < 0.001$; n.a.: not applicable.

4. Discussion

There is increasing evidence that aquatic athletes—including swimmers, water polo players, and apnea divers—consistently show superior pulmonary function when compared to athletes from non-aquatic sports such as football or basketball [11,12]. Their lungs can withstand greater transpulmonary volumes and pressures than the average population, likely due to a combination of genetic predisposition and structural adaptations resulting from repeated pulmonary distension [8,12]. However, it is known that although water polo players exhibited elevated FEV1 and FVC values, their FEV1/FVC ratio was lower, possibly indicating either reduced ventilatory efficiency or greater functional residual capacity [12]. Likewise, spirometric findings in BWS reveal a mean FEV1/FVC ratio of 76.19 ± 6.17%, bordering on the threshold for obstructive impairment. In addition, reduced $FEF_{25-75\%}$ values were found in 64.7% of BWS, suggesting potential small airway impairment, as observed in individuals performing lung packing or repeated glossopharyngeal insufflation (GPB) [13]. Big Wave Surfers also demonstrated significantly elevated maximal inspiratory (MIP = 138.35 ± 29.03 cmH_2O) and expiratory (MEP = 143.88 ± 27.89 cmH_2O) pressures when compared to untrained individuals (MIP = 115.29 ± 24.98 cmH_2O; MEP = 118.33 ± 23.5 cmH_2O) [12] and apnea divers (MIP = 131.30 ± 24.98 cmH_2O; MEP = 132 ± 30.01 cmH_2O) [5]. This is probably due to the fact that apnea training causes an increase in respiratory workload, since the hydrostatic forces to which the individual is subjected compress and deform the thorax, requiring the inspiratory muscles to counteract these forces, which leads to deeper inspirations and longer respiratory cycles. Apnea training causes an increase in respiratory workload, since the hydrostatic forces to which the individual is subjected compress and deform the thorax, requiring the inspiratory muscles to counteract these forces. This leads to deeper inspirations and longer respiratory cycles [14]. As for GPB, besides being an important training strategy to deal with hypoxic stress during apnea [15], it can lead to respiratory muscle dysfunction due to strenuous training and continuous demand on the respiratory muscles [4] and to a significant reduction in the elastic component of the lungs [7]. Given the repetitive and forceful nature of apnea during wipeouts, and the significant compressive forces experienced underwater, BWS may be at risk for chronic pulmonary changes. Therefore, further longitudinal studies are warranted to evaluate potential health risks, including obstructive lung disease, impaired diffusion capacity, and pulmonary hypertension, like those documented in divers [16]. Apnea training and accumulated years of exposure likely benefit BWS by inducing physiological adaptations that reduce CO_2 sensitivity and delay involuntary respiratory muscle contractions during breath-holding, thereby improving hypoxia tolerance. On the other hand, repeated apnea episodes and associated techniques like GPB may alter thoracic shape and the respiratory muscle mechanics, paralleling adaptations observed in chronic obstructive pulmonary disease. This ventilatory pattern may predispose BWS to decreased pulmonary compliance and increase the risk of barotrauma, pneumomediastinum, and chronic pulmonary dysfunction.

As an unstudied population, this research provides the first insights into the respiratory profile of BWS, addressing spirometric characterization and the identification of functional adaptations.

5. Conclusions

The athletes assessed exhibit enhanced respiratory function when compared to the general population, sharing several physiological features with swimmers and apnea divers, such as increased ventilatory capacity (FVC, PEF, MIP, and MEP). However, their FEV1/FVC ratio hovers around 70%, which may signal potential obstructive airway conditions, requiring further investigation.

Author Contributions: Conceptualization, P.S. and L.C.e.S.; methodology, P.S., A.L.-R.-V. and L.C.e.S.; software, P.S.; validation, P.S., A.L.-R.-V. and L.C.e.S.; formal analysis, P.S. and L.C.e.S.; investigation, P.S. and L.C.e.S.; resources, P.S. and L.C.e.S.; data curation, P.S. and A.L.-R.-V.; writing—original draft preparation, P.S.; writing—review and editing, P.S., A.L.-R.-V. and L.C.e.S.; supervision, P.S. All authors have read and agreed to the published version of the manuscript.

Funding: This research received no external funding.

Institutional Review Board Statement: The study was conducted in accordance with the Declaration of Helsinki and approved by the Ethics Committee of ESCOLA SUPERIOR DE SAÚDE ATLÂNTICA (PCE05_2022) for studies involving humans.

Informed Consent Statement: It was obtained from all subjects involved in the study.

Data Availability Statement: The data presented in this study are available on request from the corresponding author due to the General Data Protection Rules.

Acknowledgments: The authors would like to acknowledge the CAR NAZARÉ staff for providing access to the facilities to conduct the study and ESSATLA for providing the needed materials.

Conflicts of Interest: The authors declare no conflicts of interest.

References

1. Farrell, T. Big wave surfing—A physician's perspective. *Sports Orthop. Traumatol.* **2018**, *34*, 253–255. [CrossRef]
2. Farley, O.; Abbiss, C.; Sheppard, J. Testing protocols for profiling of surfers' anaerobic and aerobic fitness: A review. *Strength. Cond. J.* **2016**, *38*, 52–65. [CrossRef]
3. Lazovic, B.; Mazic, S.; Suzic-Lazic, J.; Djelic, M.; Djordjevic-Saranovic, S.; Durmic, T.; Zikic, D.; Zugic, V. Respiratory adaptation in different types of sport. *Eur. Rev. Med. Pharmacol. Sci.* **2015**, *19*, 2269–2274. [PubMed]
4. Tetzlaff, K.; Scholz, T.; Walterspacher, S.; Muth, C.; Metzger, J.; Roecker, K.; Sorichter, S. Characteristics of the respiratory mechanical and muscle function of competitive breath-hold divers. *Eur. J. Appl. Physiol.* **2008**, *103*, 469–475. [CrossRef] [PubMed]
5. Diniz, C.; Farias, T.; Pereira, M.; Pires, C.; Gonçalves, L.; Coertjens, P.; Coertjens, M. Chronic adaptations of lung function in breath-hold diving fishermen. *Int. J. Occup. Med. Environ. Health* **2014**, *27*, 216–223. [CrossRef] [PubMed]
6. Rochat, I.; Côté, A.; Boulet, L. Determinants of lung function changes in athletic swimmers. A review. *Acta Paediatr.* **2021**, *111*, 259–264. [CrossRef] [PubMed]
7. Chung, S.; Seccombe, L.; Jenkins, C.; Frater, C.; Ridley, L.; Peters, M. Glossopharyngeal insufflation causes lung injury in trained breath-hold divers. *Respirology* **2010**, *15*, 813–817. [CrossRef] [PubMed]
8. Loring, S.; O'Donnell, C.; Butler, J.; Lindholm, P.; Jacobson, F.; Ferrigno, M. Transpulmonary pressures and lung mechanics with glossopharyngeal insufflation and exsufflation beyond normal lung volumes in competitive breath-hold divers. *J. Appl. Physiol.* **2007**, *102*, 841–846. [CrossRef] [PubMed]
9. Fritz-Clarke, J. Breath-Hold diving. *Compr. Physiol.* **2018**, *8*, 585–630. [CrossRef]
10. Graham, B.; Steenbruggen, I.; Miller, M.; Barjaktarevic, I.; Cooper, B.; Hall, G.; Hallstrand, T.; Kaminsky, D.; McCarthy, K.; McCormack, M.; et al. Standardization of Spirometry 2019 Update, An Official American Thoracic Society and European Respiratory Society Technical Statement. *Am. J. Respir. Crit. Care Med.* **2019**, *200*, e70–e88. [CrossRef] [PubMed]
11. Durmic, T.; Lazovic, B.; Djelic, M.; Lazic, J.; Zikic, D.; Zugic, V.; Dekleva, M.; Mazic, S. Sport-specific influences on respiratory patterns in elite athletes. *J. Bras. Pneumol.* **2015**, *41*, 516–522. [CrossRef] [PubMed]

12. Segizbaeva, M.; Aleksandrova, N. Respiratory Muscle Strength and Ventilatory Function Outcome: Differences Between Trained Athletes and Healthy Untrained Persons. *Adv. Exp. Med. Biol.* **2021**, *1289*, 89–97. [CrossRef] [PubMed]
13. Ronish, B.; Couper, D.; Barjaktarevic, I.; Cooper, C.; Kanner, R.; Pirozzi, C.; Kim, V.; Wells, J.; Han, M.; Woodruff, P.; et al. Forced Expiratory Flow at 25%–75% Links COPD Physiology to Emphysema and Disease Severity in the SPIROMICS Cohort. *Chronic Obstr. Pulm. Dis.* **2022**, *9*, 111–121. [CrossRef]
14. Stavrou, V.; Toubekis, A.G.; Karetsi, E. Changes in Respiratory Parameters and Fin-Swimming Performance Following a 16-Week Training Period with Intermittent Breath Holding. *J. Hum. Kinet.* **2015**, *49*, 89–98. [CrossRef]
15. Lemaître, F.; Billaut, F.; Joulia, F. Editorial: Physiology and Physiopathology of Breath-Holding Activity. *Front. Physiol.* **2022**, *13*, 858371. [CrossRef] [PubMed]
16. Dujic, Z.; Breskovic, T. Impact of Breath Holding on Cardiovascular Respiratory and Cerebrovascular Health. *Sports Med.* **2012**, *42*, 459–472. [CrossRef] [PubMed]

medical sciences forum

MDPI

Proceeding Paper

Influence of Coca-Cola® on Thermoplastic Degradation in Clear Orthodontic Aligners †

Margarida Pitschieller [1], Dinis Pereira [1,2], Ana Sintra Delgado [1,2] and Carla Ascenso [1,*]

1 Egas Moniz Center for Interdisciplinary Research (CiiEM), Egas Moniz School of Health and Science, Quinta da Granja, 2829-511 Caparica, Portugal; greta.lpit@gmail.com (M.P.); dpereira@egasmoniz.edu.pt (D.P.); adelgado@egasmoniz.edu.pt (A.S.D.)

2 Clinical Research Unit (CRU), Orthodontics Department, Egas Moniz Center for Interdisciplinary Research (CiiEM), Egas Moniz School of Health and Science, 2829-511 Caparica, Portugal

* Correspondence: carla.ascenso@egasmoniz.edu.pt

† Presented at the 7th CiiEM International Congress 2025—Empowering One Health to Reduce Social Vulnerabilities, Caparica, Portugal, 2–4 July 2025.

Abstract: Clear orthodontic aligners, primarily composed of thermoplastic polymers, are increasingly popular but susceptible to degradation through thermal, chemical, and mechanical stress. This preliminary pilot study assessed the release of microplastics from two commercial aligner brands under simulated oral conditions. Aligners were exposed to daily cycles of Coca-Cola® or artificial saliva, with mechanical agitation replicating masticatory friction. Fourier-transform infrared spectroscopy confirmed microplastic release in both environments, with a notably higher particle count after Coca-Cola® exposure. These findings indicate the potential health and environmental risks linked to acidic beverage consumption during orthodontic treatment. Further comprehensive studies are required to validate and expand upon these results.

Keywords: microplastics; clear orthodontic aligners; Coca-Cola®; FTIR spectroscopy

1. Introduction

Since the introduction of clear thermoplastic orthodontic aligners by Invisalign® in 1997, their use has grown substantially due to their aesthetic and functional advantages. As removable devices, clear orthodontic aligners (COAs) require strict patient compliance to ensure effective treatment outcomes. Typically, each aligner is worn for approximately seven days, although a 14-day protocol may be necessary for complex tooth movements (e.g., torque, inclination, and rotation) [1]. After this period, the aligner is replaced by a new one. This sequence continues until the orthodontic treatment is completed. Aligners should be worn for 20–22 h per day [1], and manufacturers recommend their removal during the consumption of any food or beverages other than water and for oral hygiene procedures. Nevertheless, many patients do not adhere strictly to these guidelines, often consuming beverages or even food while wearing the aligners [2].

During use, aligners are exposed to the oral environment, which is characterised by fluctuating temperature and pH, as well as mechanical, thermal, and enzymatic challenges. These factors can compromise the structural integrity of the aligner material. Inappropriate behaviours, such as consuming acidic beverages like Coca-Cola® or fruit juices, can accelerate material degradation [3]. Previous studies have reported morphological changes in aligners after clinical use, including biofilm accumulation, microcracks, and abrasions, which may facilitate the release of microplastic particles [4,5].

Commercial aligners differ in material composition, thickness, and clinical protocols, with each brand utilising specific thermoplastic polymers such as polyurethane (PU), polyethylene terephthalate (PET), polyethylene glycol terephthalate (PETG), and polyvinyl chloride (PVC). The toxicity of plastics varies with polymer type and particle size, with smaller particles generally exhibiting higher toxicity. Microplastics (MPs), defined as particles smaller than 5 mm, and nanoplastics (NPs), smaller than 100 nm [6], have been detected in various human tissues and fluids. The European Food Safety Authority has reported that MPs/NPs smaller than 150 μm may cross the intestinal epithelium [7] and have been detected in various human tissues and fluids [8]. Existing studies suggest that the biopersistence of MPs leads to a range of immune responses including inflammation, genotoxicity, oxidative stress, apoptosis, and necrosis [8]. Given the potential for aligners to contribute to microplastic exposure, particularly when used inappropriately, it is essential to conduct further research to clarify the extent and significance of this phenomenon. This pilot study aimed to assess whether the consumption of beverages such as Coca-Cola® promotes the release of MPs by COAs compared to the results already published when only artificial saliva was used [5].

2. Materials and Methods

The experimental protocol used in this study was adapted from Quinzi et al. [5]. In total, 12 pairs of COAs (n = 24) were acquired from two different brands, Dentsply Sirona (Group A, n = 12) and Invisalign (Group B, n = 12), from different patients and not clinically used. Each group of samples was subjected to a seven-day in vitro protocol designed to simulate oral conditions. Aligners were immersed for 5 h/day in either regular Coca-Cola® (pH 2.5) or artificial saliva (pH 6.8) [9] and stirred to simulate the physiological friction produced by patient tooth movement. Following this period, the immersion medium was replaced with fresh artificial saliva, and the samples were maintained at 37 °C without stirring for the remaining 19 h/day. This cycle was repeated daily for seven days. All solutions in contact with each group of samples, including rinsing water, were collected and vacuum-filtered through 1.6 μm membranes. The retained particles were examined under a stereomicroscope and characterised by Fourier-transform infrared spectroscopy (FTIR) by contact. All FTIR spectra were obtained in the range of 4000 to 400 cm^{-1}, and 31 scans were performed per analysis. The spectra of the collected particles were compared with those of the original aligner materials to confirm the identity of the polymers.

3. Results

Both aligner brands released microplastic particles under the tested conditions, and the stereomicroscope images of some are shown in Figure 1. The number of particles released was visibly higher following exposure to Coca-Cola® compared to artificial saliva. The FTIR spectra of the as-received aligners (Figure 2, blue lines) showed the characteristic peaks for the presence of polyethylene terephthalate (PET) for the Dentsply Sirona COA, Group A; polyurethane, PU, for the Invisalign COA, Group B. FTIR analysis of the particles collected after filtration (Figure 2, dark lines) and comparison of the spectra obtained with the original COA (by correlation percentages) confirmed the presence of microplastics. No evidence of extraneous contamination was detected. The amount of MP released in the test with Coca-Cola® was always higher than in the control with artificial saliva. These results should be interpreted with caution due to the limited sample size.

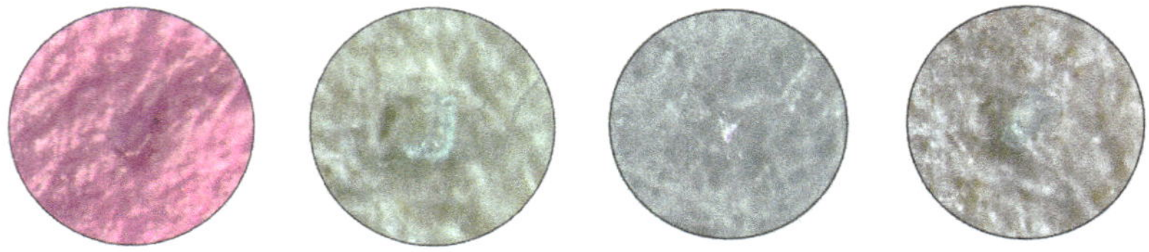

(**a**) (**b**) (**c**) (**d**)

Figure 1. Stereomicroscope images of some particles obtained after filtration: Group A tested with (**a**) artificial saliva and with (**b**) Coca-Cola; Group B tested with (**c**) artificial saliva and with (**d**) Coca-Cola.

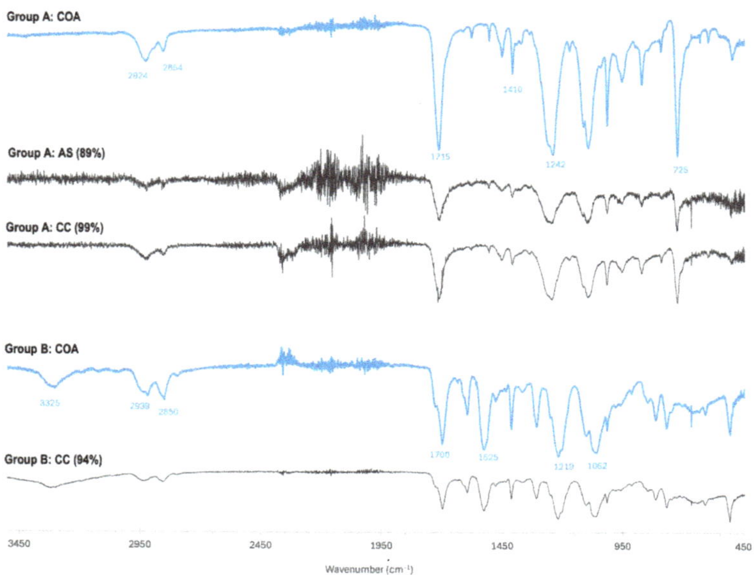

Figure 2. Comparison between the FTIR spectra of the as-received COA (in blue) with the characteristic molecular bands and the FTIR spectra of the representative collected microparticles detached from the aligners (dark lines). The percentage value in brackets refers to the correlation with the original COA. AS, artificial saliva; CC, Coca-Cola.

4. Discussion

The acidic environment produced by Coca-Cola® appears to accelerate the degradation of thermoplastic polymers used in orthodontic aligners. Repeated acid exposure, combined with mechanical friction, likely increases material fatigue and surface erosion, promoting microplastic release. These findings, although based on a small sample and in vitro simulation, raise concerns considering the growing evidence that microplastics can cross epithelial barriers, accumulate in tissues, and elicit cellular stress responses. Chronic exposure has been linked to endocrine disruption and altered immune responses, which may have systemic implications, particularly for younger patients undergoing prolonged orthodontic treatment. As a pilot study, these results reinforce existing recommendations discouraging the consumption of acidic beverages while wearing aligners and underscore the importance of further research.

5. Conclusions

This pilot study demonstrates that artificial saliva alone can induce microplastic release from orthodontic aligners, with Coca-Cola® exposure significantly increasing this effect. The results highlight the potential influence of patient behaviour on material stability and microplastic exposure. Further comprehensive studies are essential to confirm these findings, determine their clinical relevance, and guide evidence-based recommendations for orthodontic practice.

Author Contributions: Conceptualization, C.A. and D.P.; methodology, C.A. and M.P.; investigation, C.A. and M.P.; writing—original draft preparation, M.P.; writing—review and editing, C.A., D.P., and A.S.D.; supervision, C.A., D.P., and A.S.D. All authors have read and agreed to the published version of the manuscript.

Funding: This research received no external funding.

Institutional Review Board Statement: Not applicable.

Informed Consent Statement: Not applicable.

Data Availability Statement: Data are contained within the article.

Conflicts of Interest: The authors declare no conflicts of interest.

References

1. Al-Nadawi, M.; Kravitz, N.D.; Hansa, I.; Makki, L.; Ferguson, D.J.; Vaid, N.R. Effect of clear aligner wear protocol on the efficacy of tooth movement: A randomised clinical trial. *Angle Orthod.* **2021**, *91*, 157–163. [CrossRef] [PubMed]
2. Bernard, G.; Rompré, P.; Tavares, J.R.; Montpetit, A. Colorimetric and spectrophotometric measurements of orthodontic thermoplastic aligners exposed to various staining sources and cleaning methods. *Head Face Med.* **2020**, *16*, 2. [CrossRef] [PubMed]
3. Warnecki, M.; Sarul, M.; Kozakiewicz, M.; Zięty, A.; Babiarczuk, B.; Kawala, B.; Jurzysynk, Z. Surface evaluation of aligners after compulsory teeth immersion in Coca-Cola and orange juice. *Materials* **2022**, *15*, 6341. [CrossRef] [PubMed]
4. Bucci, R.; Rongo, R.; Levaté, C.; Michelotti, A.; Barone, S.; Razionale, A.V.; D'Antò, V. Thickness of orthodontic clear aligners after thermoforming and after 10 days of intraoral exposure: A prospective clinical study. *Prog. Orthod.* **2019**, *20*, 36. [CrossRef] [PubMed]
5. Quinzi, V.; Orilisi, G.; Vitiello, F.; Nofrasterino, V.; Marzo, G.; Orsini, G. A spectroscopic study on orthodontic aligners: First evidence of microplastic dispersion after seven days of clinical use. *Sci. Total Environ.* **2023**, *886*, 161356. [CrossRef] [PubMed]
6. Otorkpa, O.J.; Otorkpa, C.O. Health effects of microplastics and nanoplastics: Review of published case reports. *Environ. Anal. Health Toxicol.* **2024**, *39*, e2024020. [CrossRef]
7. Choi, H.; Kaneko, S.; Suzuki, Y.; Inamura, K.; Nishikawa, M.; Sakai, Y. Size dependent internalization of microplastics and nanoplastics using in vitro model of the human intestine—Contribution of each cell in the tri-culture models. *Nanomaterials* **2024**, *14*, 1435. [CrossRef] [PubMed]
8. Wang, X.; Deng, K.; Zhang, P.; Chen, Q.; Magnuson, J.T.; Qiu, W.; Zhou, Y. Microplastic-mediated new mechanism of liver damage: From the perspective of the gut-liver axis. *Sci. Total Environ.* **2024**, *919*, 170962. [CrossRef] [PubMed]
9. Gal, J.Y.; Fovet, Y.; Adib-Yadzi, M. About a synthetic saliva for in vitro studies. *Talanta* **2001**, *53*, 1103–1115. [CrossRef]

medical sciences forum

MDPI

Proceeding Paper

Efficacy of Topical Sialogogues in Xerostomia Treatment on Chronic Residents of C.H.P.L. †

Edna Verissimo [1,*], Cecília Rozan [1,2] and Ana Cristina Manso [1,2]

1 Instituto Universitário Egas Moniz (IUEM), Egas Moniz School of Health & Science, 2829-511 Caparica, Almada, Portugal; crozan@egasmoniz.edu.pt (C.R.); cmanso@egasmoniz.edu.pt (A.C.M.)
2 Egas Moniz Center for Interdisciplinary Research (CiiEM), Egas Moniz School of Health & Science, 2829-511 Caparica, Almada, Portugal
* Correspondence: everissimo@egasmoniz.edu.pt
† Presented at the 7th CiiEM International Congress 2025—Empowering One Health to Reduce Social Vulnerabilities, Caparica, Portugal, 2–4 July 2025.

Abstract: Institutionalized psychiatric patients on chronic psychotropic medication are prone to xerostomia due to reduced salivary flow. This study evaluated the effectiveness of a topical sialogogue gel (*Xeros Dentaid*®) in relieving drug-induced dry mouth in 81 residents at the Lisbon Psychiatric Hospital Centre (C.H.P.L.). Over 15 days, unstimulated and stimulated salivary flow rates, pH, and buffer capacity were measured before and after application. Results showed a significant increase in salivary flow ($p < 0.001$) and improved subjective symptoms. Topical sialogogues may represent an accessible and effective strategy for managing xerostomia in this vulnerable population.

Keywords: psychotic disorders; hyposialia; xerostomia

1. Introduction

Xerostomia, the subjective sensation of oral dryness, is a common adverse effect of chronic pharmacotherapy, particularly among institutionalized psychiatric patients receiving antipsychotics and anticholinergic agents [1]. The reduction in salivary flow, known as hyposialia, has been shown to impair essential oral functions such as lubrication, antimicrobial defense and remineralization, which can increase the risk of caries, mucosal infections, and reduced quality of life [2]. This population is especially vulnerable due to polypharmacy and limited access to preventive dental care [1]. Topical sialogogues present a promising therapeutic alternative by virtue of their capacity to locally stimulate salivary flow with minimal systemic side effects. Nevertheless, the clinical evidence supporting their use in this specific context remains limited [3,4]. The objective of this study is to evaluate the effectiveness of a topical sialogogue gel in improving salivary flow and relieving symptoms of xerostomia (dry mouth) in long-term residents of the Lisbon Psychiatric Hospital Centre (C.H.P.L.). The findings of this study will contribute to the development strategies to improve oral health in individuals with complex medical conditions and high social vulnerability.

2. Materials and Methods

A cross-sectional, correlational study was conducted from March to June 2023 over a period of four months at the Lisbon Psychiatric Hospital Centre (C.H.P.L.), involving three closed psychiatric inpatient wards (18, 21B, and Forensic ward). The study was approved by the Scientific and Pedagogical Committee and the Ethics Committee of the C.H.P.L., as well as by the hospital's Executive Board (approval number: 1197). All participants were informed of the study objectives and procedures and provided written informed consent, in accordance with the Declaration of Helsinki and national legislation.

A total of 81 institutionalized patients with chronic psychiatric conditions who met the inclusion criteria and voluntarily agreed to participate were enrolled. The inclusion criteria comprised the following: (1) age $\geq$ 18 years; (2) permanent inpatient status at C.H.P.L.; (3) both sexes; and (4) capacity to understand and sign informed consent. Salivary flow was assessed using sialometry at baseline (T0) and after 15 days (T1). A subsequent investigation involved the implementation of a questionnaire regarding sociodemographic variables and the *Summated Xerostomia Inventory*—Portuguese short version (SXI-PL). The unstimulated salivary flow rate (USFR) was measured via passive drooling; the stimulated salivary flow rate (SSFR) was collected by chewing a 1g sterile paraffin tablet. Buffer capacity and pH were evaluated using *Saliva Check-buffer*® kits. Hyposialia was defined as USFR < 0.1 mL/min and/or SSFR < 0.7 mL/min. Participants received topical application of *Xeros Dentaid Gel*® (betaine 1%, aloe vera 0.05%, xylitol 10%, sodium fluoride 0.0033%), administered by trained nurses two times a day, after oral hygiene and before main meals, for 15 consecutive days. The application covered teeth, gingivae, and oral floor without rinsing, ensuring optimal overnight hydration. Data were analyzed using IBM SPSS Statistics® v.28.

3. Results

A total of 81 institutionalized psychiatric patients participated in the study, with a mean age of 47.83 $\pm$ 15.39 years. Most participants were male (81.5%, n = 66), with only 18.5% (n = 15) identifying as female. The frequency distributions of psychiatric patients were as follows: schizophrenia and schizotypal and delusional disorders, 59.2% (48); epilepsy, 21% (17); and neurotic, stress-related, and somatoform disorders, 16 (19.8%). The majority of patients in the study were medicated with antipsychotics (98.8% (80)) and antiepileptics (55.6% (45)), followed by anxiolytics (72.8% (59)), antidepressants (43.2% (35)), and hypnotics/sedatives (28.4% (23)).

3.1. Salivary Flow Rates—Before and After Treatment

The unstimulated salivary flow rate (USFR) at baseline (T0) ranged from 0 to 3 mL/min, with a mean of 0.43 $\pm$ 0.47 mL/min. The stimulated salivary flow rate (SSFR) at T0 ranged from 0 to 3 mL/min, with a mean of 0.53 $\pm$ 0.58 mL/min. Fifteen days after topical sialogogue application (T1), USFR increased to 0.72 $\pm$ 0.54 mL/min and SSFR to 0.69 $\pm$ 0.68 mL/min. The mean increases of 0.28 mL/min in USFR and 0.15 mL/min in SSFR were statistically significant ($p < 0.001$), suggesting clear improvement in salivary function following treatment.

3.2. Prevalence of Xerostomia/Hyposialia

At baseline (T0), 13 patients (16%) were classified as having hyposialia (USFR < 0.1 mL/min and/or SSFR < 0.7 mL/min), while 68 (84%) presented normal salivary flow (Table 1). After 15 days of treatment (T1), the prevalence of xerostomia dropped to 7.4% (n = 6), while 92.6% (n = 75) exhibited normal salivary flow (Table 2). Fisher's Exact Test confirmed a statistically significant difference in xerostomia prevalence before and after treatment ($p < 0.001$), demonstrating the efficacy of the topical sialogogue in reducing drug-induced xerostomia among psychiatric inpatients (Figure 1).

Table 1. Distribution of the frequency among salivary flow conditions (T0).

Salivary Flow Status at Baseline (T0)	Absolute Frequency (*n*)	Relative Frequency (%)
Normal	68	84%
Hyposialia/Xerostomia	13	16%

Table 2. Distribution of the frequency among salivary flow conditions (T1).

Salivary Flow Status After Treatment (T1)	Absolute Frequency (*n*)	Relative Frequency (%)
Normal	75	92.6%
Hyposialia/Xerostomia	6	7.4%

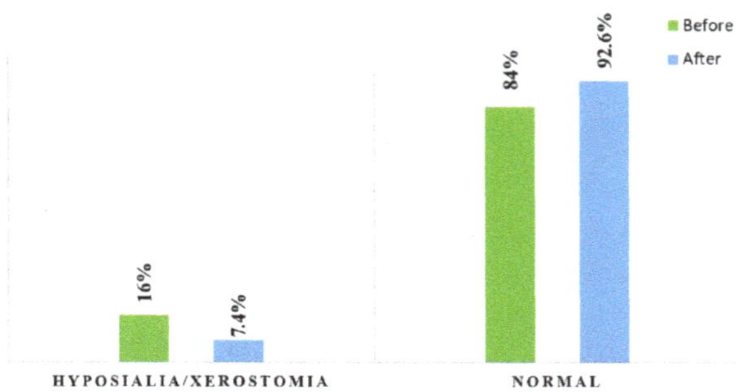

Figure 1. Distribution of xerostomia prevalence before and after treatment.

3.3. *Salivary pH and Buffer Capacity*

Although a significant increase in salivary pH was observed post-intervention (Tables 3 and 4), no significant alterations were noted in buffer capacity. These findings suggest that while the sialogogue improves hydration and flow, it does not modify the intrinsic buffering properties of saliva.

Table 3. Descriptive analysis of salivary pH assessment at baseline (T0).

pH (T0)	Absolute Frequency (*n*)	Relative Frequency (%)
5–5.8	54	66.3%
6–6.6	17	21.3%
6.8–7.8	10	12.4%

Table 4. Descriptive analysis of salivary pH after treatment (T1).

pH (T1)	Absolute Frequency (*n*)	Relative Frequency (%)
5–5.8	44	55%
6–6.6	21	25%
6.8–7.8	16	20%

3.4. *SXI-PL*

The SXI-PL questionnaire revealed total scores ranging from 5 to 15, with a mean of 7.16 ± 2.46. A strong positive correlation was observed between total SXI-PL scores and responses to the standard dry mouth question ($p < 0.001$), confirming the internal consistency and validity of the instrument. The most frequently reported symptom was "My lips feel dry" (mean = 1.50 ± 0.65), indicating it as the most impactful in participants' perception of xerostomia (Table 5). Over half of the sample (53.1%) reported experiencing dry mouth, and these individuals had higher SXI-PL scores (mean = 8.84 ± 2.28), suggesting greater symptom severity. A statistically significant association ($p > 0.05$) was observed between antidepressant use and the presence of xerostomia, suggesting a potential contributory role of this pharmacological group in salivary flow reduction.

Table 5. Distribution of mean scores of *Summated Xerostomia Inventory* (SXI-PL).

SXI-PL	Mean	SD
My mouth feels dry when eating a meal	1.47	0.65
My mouth feels dry	1.47	0.85
I have difficulty in eating dry foods	1.36	0.57
I have difficulty swallowing certain foods	1.36	0.59
My lips feel dry	1.50	0.65
Total	7.16	2.46

4. Discussion

This study demonstrated significant improvement in both unstimulated and stimulated salivary flow rates following the application of a topical sialogogue over a 15-day period in institutionalized psychiatric patients. The mean increase in USFR and in SSFR was statistically significant ($p < 0.001$), aligning with the findings of Gómez-Moreno et al. (2013), Marín et al. (2021), and Niklander et al. (2018), who reported similar benefits from topical agents [3–5]. The prevalence of xerostomia and hyposialia decreased from 16% at baseline to 7.4% post-treatment, suggesting that even short-term use of a topical sialogogue may effectively reduce symptoms. These results reinforce evidence from Dalodom et al. (2016), although their study applied the intervention for a longer period (1 month), indicating that treatment duration may influence therapeutic outcomes [6]. The SXI-PL results showed a mean score of 7.16 ± 2.46. The item "my lips feel dry" had the highest impact (1.50 ± 0.65), indicating greater perceived severity. This finding aligns with that of Farsi (2007), who identified dry lips as the most common symptom of oral dryness, reported by 37.5% of participants [7]. Salivary pH showed a significant shift towards normal physiological values, indicating a less acidic oral environment after treatment. However, no substantial change was observed in buffer capacity, diverging from some previous studies. This difference may be attributed to the relatively short duration of the current intervention. It is evident that no adverse events were reported by the patients. Following the administration of the treatment, no clinically significant alterations were identified, and no adverse events were documented.

5. Conclusions

This study's limitations include a convenience sample, limited follow-up, and indirect administration of the gel by nursing staff. Nonetheless, the significant improvements observed highlight the potential role of topical sialogogues in xerostomia management for vulnerable populations. Future research should aim for longer-term evaluations, the integration of patient-reported outcomes, and broader population samples to consolidate these preliminary findings and guide clinical protocols in psychiatric settings.

Author Contributions: Conceptualization, E.V. and C.R.; methodology, E.V. and C.R.; software, E.V.; validation, E.V., C.R. and A.C.M.; formal analysis, E.V. and C.R.; investigation, E.V. and C.R.; resources, E.V.; data curation, E.V. and C.R.; writing—original draft preparation, E.V.; writing—review and editing, E.V., C.R. and A.C.M.; visualization, E.V., C.R. and A.C.M.; supervision, E.V. and C.R.; project administration, E.V., C.R. and A.C.M. All authors have read and agreed to the published version of the manuscript.

Funding: This research received no external funding.

Institutional Review Board Statement: The study was conducted in accordance with the Declaration of Helsinki and approved by the Ethics Committee of Egas Moniz School of Health and Science (protocol code 1197, approved in 2 March 2023).

Informed Consent Statement: Informed consent was obtained from all subjects involved in the study.

Data Availability Statement: The data presented in this study are available on request from the corresponding author. The data are not publicly available as they are part of an ongoing study.

Acknowledgments: The authors thank the outpatients who participated in the study. We are indebted to the occupational therapy and nursing staff at the CHPL.

Conflicts of Interest: The authors declare no conflicts of interest.

References

1. Carmona-Huerta, J.; Castiello-de Obeso, S.; Ramírez-Palomino, J.; Duran-Gutiérrez, R.; Cardona-Muller, D.; Grover-Paez, F.; Fernández-Dorantes, P.; Medina-Dávalos, R. Polypharmacy in a hospitalized psychiatric population: Risk estimation and damage quantification. *BMC Psychiatry* **2019**, *19*, 78. [CrossRef] [PubMed]
2. Niklander, S.; Veas, L.; Barrera, C.; Fuentes, F.; Chiappini, G.; Marshall, M. Risk factors, hyposalivation and impact of xerostomia on oral health-related quality of life. *Braz. Oral Res.* **2017**, *31*, e14. [CrossRef]
3. Gómez-Moreno, G.; Guardia, J.; Aguilar-Salvatierra, A.; Cabrera-Ayala, M.; de-Val, J.E.M.S.; Calvo-Guirado, J.L. Effectiveness of malic acid 1% in patients with xerostomia induced by antihypertensive drugs. *Med. Oral Patol. Oral Cir. Bucal* **2013**, *18*, e49. [CrossRef] [PubMed]
4. Marín, C.; Díaz-de-Valdés, L.; Conejeros, C.; Martínez, R.; Niklander, S. Interventions for the treatment of xerostomia: A randomized controlled clinical trial. *J. Clin. Exp. Dent.* **2021**, *13*, e104–e111. [CrossRef] [PubMed]
5. Niklander, S.; Fuentes, F.; Sanchez, D.; Araya, V.; Chiappini, G.; Martinez, R.; Marshall, M. Impact of 1% malic acid spray on the oral health-related quality of life of patients with xerostomia. *J. Oral Sci.* **2018**, *60*, 278–284. [CrossRef] [PubMed]
6. Dalodom, S.; Lam-Ubol, A.; Jeanmaneechotechai, S.; Takamfoo, L.; Intachai, W.; Duangchada, K.; Hongsachum, B.; Kanjanatiwat, P.; Vacharotayangul, P.; Trachootham, D. Influence of oral moisturizing jelly as a saliva substitute for the relief of xerostomia in elderly patients with hypertension and diabetes mellitus. *Geriatr. Nurs.* **2016**, *37*, 101–109. [CrossRef] [PubMed]
7. Farsi, N.M. Signs of oral dryness in relation to salivary flow rate, pH, buffering capacity and dry mouth complaints. *BMC Oral Health* **2007**, *7*, 15. [CrossRef] [PubMed]

medical sciences forum

MDPI

Proceeding Paper

Patient Awareness and Acceptance of Laser Technology in Endodontics: A Cross-Sectional Study †

Marta Alves Duarte [1,2,*], João Albernaz Neves [1,3] and Javier Flores-Fraile [2]

[1] Instituto Universitário Egas Moniz, Egas Moniz School of Health & Science, 2829-511 Almada, Portugal; jalbernaz@egasmoniz.edu.pt
[2] Escuela de Doctorado Studii Salamantini, Universidad de Salamanca, 37008 Salamanca, Spain; j.flores@usal.es
[3] Egas Moniz Center for Interdisciplinary Research (CiiEM), Egas Moniz School of Health & Science, 2829-511 Almada, Portugal
* Correspondence: mduarte@egasmoniz.edu.pt
† Presented at the 7th CiiEM International Congress 2025—Empowering One Health to Reduce Social Vulnerabilities, Caparica, Portugal, 2–4 July 2025.

Abstract: Laser technology is becoming an essential part of endodontic practice due to its clear clinical advantages. A cross-sectional survey of 501 participants found that, although awareness remains limited, the results suggest that patients are willing to trust and accept laser-based treatments when recommended by dentists. In addition to the benefits of improved precision, reduced discomfort and superior disinfection, the use of lasers also promotes a sense of safety and confidence. These findings emphasise the importance of improving public understanding of, and support for, the integration of laser technology into modern dental care, since patient acceptance is essential for wider implementation.

Keywords: laser; endodontic treatment; clinical acceptance; dentistry

1. Introduction

The primary objectives of endodontic therapy are the eradication of bacteria and the elimination of microbial biofilms within the root canal system [1]. Achieving effective disinfection remains a significant clinical challenge, particularly in complex anatomical areas where conventional instrumentation and irrigation may be insufficient [2]. In this context, laser-activated irrigation has emerged as a promising adjunctive technique [3], specifically designed to enhance the penetration and efficacy of irrigating solutions during root canal treatment [4,5].

Laser-assisted protocols have been shown to improve clinical outcomes by increasing the antimicrobial effect [6], facilitating the removal of the smear layer [7], and promoting more effective cleaning of intricately shaped canals [8]. Depending on the laser type and settings used, additional benefits may include stimulation of tissue healing and regeneration, thereby contributing to long-term treatment success [6]. Moreover, the application of laser technology in endodontics may reduce postoperative discomfort [9,10] and shorten treatment time, offering both clinicians and patients a more predictable and efficient therapeutic approach [5].

Given its capacity to access areas that are often unreachable by traditional methods and its potential to significantly enhance disinfection protocols [11], the integration of lasers into routine endodontic practice warrants careful consideration [12]. However, despite these potential benefits, the perceptions, awareness, and emotional responses of patients regarding laser use in endodontic treatment remain underexplored. Understanding patients' receptiveness to such innovations is essential for guiding clinical decision-making and improving the overall patient experience.

2. Materials and Methods

This study was conducted among 503 individuals, of whom only 501 responses were considered valid, as 2 participants did not complete the questionnaire. Inclusion criteria comprised patients residing in the Lisbon district who had previously attended at least one dental appointment, while dental practitioners were excluded from participation. The anonymous questionnaire aimed to assess patients' knowledge, perceptions, and understanding of the implications of laser use in endodontics, as well as to evaluate their receptiveness to such treatment and the emotions it evokes. Data collection was carried out via Google Forms between January and May 2025.

3. Results and Discussion

A total of 503 individuals participated in the study, of which 501 responses were deemed valid; 2 were excluded due to incomplete questionnaire submissions. The most common age group among respondents was 20–30 years, followed by the 40–50-year age group. With regard to gender distribution, 52.1% of participants identified as male and 47.7% as female, while 0.2% preferred not to disclose their gender (Figure 1).

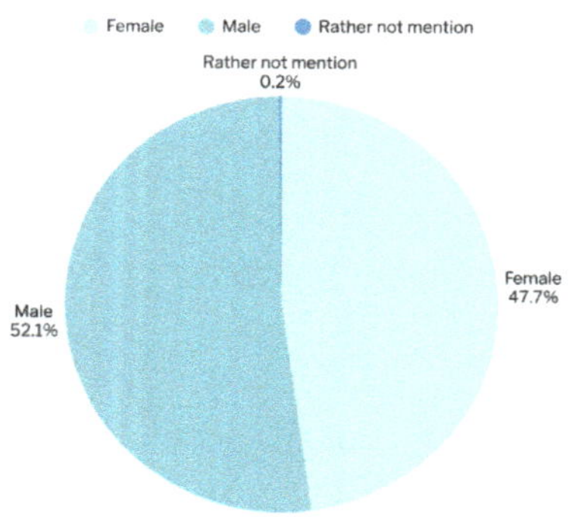

Figure 1. Gender distribution of the study participants: 52.1% identified as male, 47.7% as female, and 0.2% preferred not to disclose their gender.

Overall, 61.4% of respondents were aware that lasers can be utilised in medical/dental procedures. Additionally, 66.6% reported having undergone at least one endodontic treatment in the past. However, a substantial majority, 95.8%, had never received any form of dental treatment involving the use of laser technology.

Participants were also asked how they would react upon learning that their dental treatment would involve the use of a laser. The majority, 62.1%, stated that they would feel confident in their dentist, while 30.3% reported feeling curious, 4.0% enthusiastic, and 2.4% expressed doubt but would still accept the treatment. Only 1.2% indicated that they would feel apprehensive (Figure 2).

When questioned about their response if a dentist specifically recommended the use of lasers in endodontic therapy, 51.3% stated they would accept the treatment without hesitation, whereas 46.9% would agree but would prefer to receive further explanation beforehand and 1.8% would look for a second opinion (Figure 3).

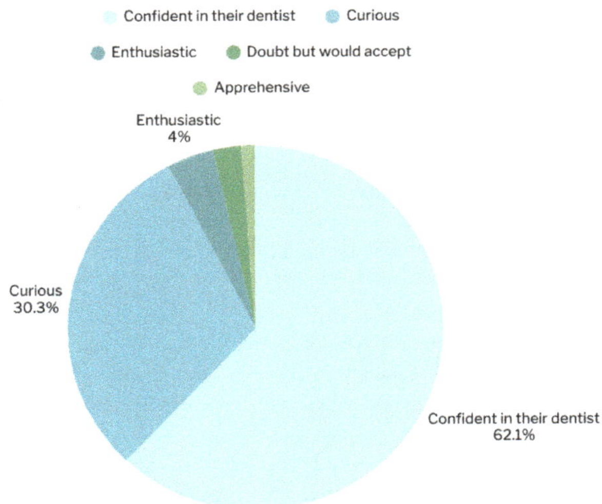

Figure 2. Participants' emotional responses to the prospect of undergoing dental treatment involving laser technology. The majority (62.1%) reported confidence, followed by curiosity (30.3%), enthusiasm (4.0%), doubt (2.4%), and apprehension (1.2%).

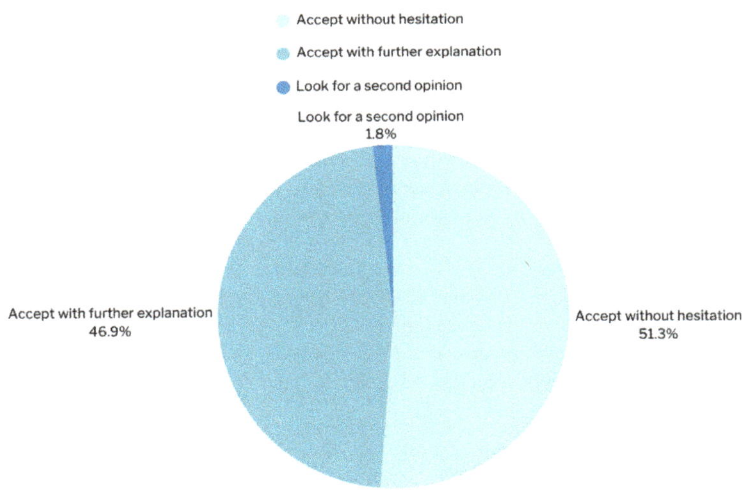

Figure 3. Willingness of participants to accept laser-assisted endodontic treatment if recommended by a dentist. Over half (51.3%) would accept without hesitation, while 46.9% would accept after receiving further explanation, and 1.8% would seek a second opinion.

The findings of this study suggest several important conclusions regarding patients' awareness, previous exposure, and receptiveness to the use of laser technology in endodontic procedures. Although a substantial proportion of participants, 61.4%, reported being aware that lasers can be utilised in dental treatments, the vast majority, 95.8%, indicated that they had never undergone any dental procedure involving the use of laser technology. This discrepancy highlights a limited clinical application or visibility of laser-based treatments within the surveyed population, despite moderate general awareness.

Notably, patients demonstrated a predominantly positive attitude towards the potential use of lasers in their own dental care. When asked how they would react if informed that their treatment would involve laser technology, most respondents expressed confidence in their dentist, 62.1%, or curiosity, 30.3%, or enthusiasm, 4%. Only a small minority reported doubt, 2.4%, or apprehension, 1.2%. These findings suggest a high level of receptiveness to laser-assisted treatments, provided that patients are informed and trust their clinician.

Furthermore, when presented with a hypothetical recommendation by their dentist to use a laser in endodontic therapy, 51.3% of participants stated they would accept the treatment without hesitation, while 46.9% would agree but expressed a desire for further explanation. This underscores the critical role of effective patient–practitioner communication, particularly when introducing technologies that may be unfamiliar to the general public.

4. Conclusions

Laser technology is increasingly becoming a part of contemporary clinical dental practice, and the results of this study suggest that patients generally welcome its integration.

Although direct experience with laser-assisted procedures remains limited among the population surveyed, the overall attitude was markedly positive. Most respondents expressed either trust in their dentist or curiosity when presented with the idea of laser use in endodontics, with only a very small proportion indicating doubt or apprehension. Furthermore, over half of the participants would accept laser treatment without hesitation if recommended by their dentist, while nearly all others would accept it with additional explanation—highlighting the key role of communication in facilitating acceptance of new technologies.

These findings underscore the potential of laser technology not only as a clinical tool but also as a means of enhancing the patient experience. In fact, the use of advanced technology appears to instill greater confidence in patients regarding the treatments they receive, reinforcing the perception of competence and innovation in dental care. As such, its broader implementation may contribute to increased patient satisfaction and perceived quality of care. Future research should focus on identifying barriers to its routine use in dental practice, as well as evaluating long-term clinical outcomes and patient-reported experiences associated with laser-based endodontic treatments.

Author Contributions: Conceptualization, M.A.D.; methodology, M.A.D.; validation, M.A.D., J.A.N. and J.F.-F.; formal analysis, M.A.D.; investigation, M.A.D.; resources, M.A.D.; data curation, M.A.D., J.A.N. and J.F.-F.; writing—original draft preparation, M.A.D.; writing—review and editing M.A.D., J.A.N. and J.F.-F.; visualisation, M.A.D.; supervision, M.A.D. and J.A.N. and J.F.-F.; project administration, M.A.D.; funding acquisition, M.A.D. All authors have read and agreed to the published version of the manuscript.

Funding: This research received no external funding.

Institutional Review Board Statement: This study was conducted in accordance with the ethical principles of the Declaration of Helsinki and was approved by the University of Salamanca as part of the CD309748 PhD research project (1 October 2024) in Salamanca, Spain.

Informed Consent Statement: Informed consent was obtained from all subjects involved in the study.

Data Availability Statement: The original data presented in the study are openly available in Zenodo, at https://doi.org/10.5281/zenodo.15728287 (accessed on 28 August 2025).

Conflicts of Interest: The authors declare no conflicts of interest.

References

1. Tonini, R.; Salvadori, M.; Audino, E.; Sauro, S.; Garo, M.L.; Salgarello, S. Irrigating Solutions and Activation Methods Used in Clinical Endodontics: A Systematic Review. *Front. Oral Health* **2022**, 3, 838043. [CrossRef]

2. Kimura, Y.; Wilder-Smith, P.; Matsumoto, K. Lasers in endodontics: A review. *Int. Endod. J.* **2000**, *33*, 173–185. [CrossRef] [PubMed]
3. Meire, M.A.; Bronzato, J.D.; Bomfim, R.A.; Gomes, B.P.F.A. Effectiveness of adjunct therapy for the treatment of apical periodontitis: A systematic review and meta-analysis. *Int. Endod. J.* **2023**, *56*, 455–474. [CrossRef] [PubMed]
4. Anagnostaki, E.; Mylona, V.; Parker, S.; Lynch, E.; Grootveld, M. Systematic Review on the Role of Lasers in Endodontic Therapy: Valuable Adjunct Treatment? *Dent. J.* **2020**, *8*, 63. [CrossRef] [PubMed]
5. Boutsioukis, C.; Arias-Moliz, M.T. Present status and future directions—Irrigants and irrigation methods. *Int. Endod. J.* **2022**, *55* (Suppl. S3), 588–612. [CrossRef] [PubMed]
6. Ribeiro, L.; Fischer, B.V.; Vitali, F.C.; Santos, P.S.; Teixeira, C.d.S.; Queiroz, Í.O.d.A.; Sivieri-Araujo, G.; dos Santos, P.H.; Garcia, L.d.F.R. Advances in laser-assisted regenerative endodontic procedures: A scoping review. *J. Dent.* **2025**, *158*, 105783. [CrossRef] [PubMed]
7. Guidotti, R.; Merigo, E.; Fornaini, C.; Rocca, J.-P.; Medioni, E.; Vescovi, P. Er:YAG 2,940-nm laser fiber in endodontic treatment: A help in removing smear layer. *Lasers Med. Sci.* **2014**, *29*, 69–75. [CrossRef] [PubMed]
8. Liapis, D.; De Bruyne, M.A.A.; De Moor, R.J.G.; Meire, M.A. Postoperative pain after ultrasonically and laser-activated irrigation during root canal treatment: A randomized clinical trial. *Int. Endod. J.* **2021**, *54*, 1037–1050. [CrossRef] [PubMed]
9. Huang, Q.; Li, Z.; Lyu, P.; Zhou, X.; Fan, Y. Current Applications and Future Directions of Lasers in Endodontics: A Narrative Review. *Bioengineering* **2023**, *10*, 296. [CrossRef] [PubMed]
10. Sen, O.G.; Kaya, M. Effect of Root Canal Disinfection with a Diode Laser on Postoperative Pain After Endodontic Retreatment. *Photobiomodul. Photomed. Laser Surg.* **2019**, *37*, 85–90. [CrossRef]
11. Morsy, D.A.; Negm, M.; Diab, A.; Ahmed, G. Postoperative pain and antibacterial effect of 980 nm diode laser versus conventional endodontic treatment in necrotic teeth with chronic periapical lesions: A randomized control trial. *F1000Research* **2018**, *7*, 1795. [CrossRef] [PubMed]
12. Pandiyan, R.; Lehl, G.K.; Kumar, R.; Sharma, U.; Jagachandiran, V.V. Assessing the efficacy of Laser pulpotomy versus conventional pulpotomy in primary teeth: A systematic review and meta-analysis of clinical trials. *Lasers Med. Sci.* **2024**, *39*, 198. [CrossRef] [PubMed]

medical sciences forum

MDPI

Proceeding Paper

Assessment of the Diagnostic Delay in a Portuguese Population of Patients with Burning Mouth Syndrome—A Preliminary Study †

Mariana Vallera Machete *, José Grillo Evangelista, Luís Proença, Pedro Ferreira Trancoso, António Mano Azul and Carlos Zagalo *

Egas Moniz Center for Interdisciplinary Research (CiiEM), Egas Moniz School of Health & Science, 2829-511 Caparica, Almada, Portugal; jgrillo@egasmoniz.edu.pt (J.G.E.); lproenca@egasmoniz.edu.pt (L.P.); ptrancoso@egasmoniz.edu.pt (P.F.T.); antonio.azul@zonmail.pt (A.M.A.)

* Correspondence: mcmachete@egasmoniz.edu.pt (M.V.M.); czagalo1@gmail.com (C.Z.); Tel.: +351-910863676 (M.V.M.)

† Presented at the 7th CiiEM International Congress 2025—Empowering One Health to Reduce Social Vulnerabilities, Caparica, Portugal, 2–4 July 2025.

Abstract: Burning Mouth Syndrome (BMS) presents diagnostic and therapeutic challenges due to its unclear etiology and complex symptomatology. This study, part of a doctoral research project, explores diagnostic delay, triggering factors, and psychotropic medication use in BMS patients. By retrospectively analyzing 300 clinical records, the study offers insight into patterns of diagnosis and treatment, with a focus on differences related to age and sex. The findings contribute to a better understanding of BMS and emphasize the need for timely diagnosis, particularly in older adults, to improve patient outcomes.

Keywords: Burning Mouth Syndrome; diagnostic delay; psychotropic medication

1. Introduction

Burning Mouth Syndrome (BMS) is a chronic orofacial pain condition characterized by a persistent or recurrent burning sensation of the oral mucosa, occurring in the absence of clinically evident lesions or laboratory abnormalities [1]. The condition predominantly affects women, particularly during peri- and postmenopausal periods, and is frequently accompanied by xerostomia, dysgeusia, and paraesthetic symptoms [2]. BMS significantly impairs quality of life, contributing to psychological distress, functional limitations, and social isolation [3].

Despite increased clinical awareness, BMS remains a diagnostic challenge. The diagnosis is fundamentally one of exclusion, necessitating the elimination of local, systemic, and psychological factors [4]. This complexity contributes to a notable diagnostic delay, with reported averages ranging from one to three years in various populations [5–7]. During this period, patients often seek multiple appointments with different doctors, undergo unnecessary investigations, and receive inappropriate treatments, which can exacerbate psychological and physical distress [5].

The etiology of BMS is multifactorial, with contributions from peripheral and central neuropathic mechanisms, hormonal fluctuations, and psychosocial factors [1,4]. Psychiatric comorbidities such as anxiety and depression are frequently reported, and the empirical prescription of psychotropic medications is common in clinical management [4]. Stress is also frequently identified as a precipitating or aggravating factor [6]. Emerging evidence suggests that age, education level, and previous psychiatric history may be predictive of longer diagnostic delays [7].

Given the significant burden of BMS and the implications of diagnostic delay on treatment outcomes, this study aims to characterize diagnostic delays and associated clinical features—including psychotropic drug use and patient-reported triggers—within a Portuguese cohort. This work forms part of a broader doctoral research project.

2. Materials and Methods

A retrospective analysis was conducted using clinical records from 300 patients diagnosed with primary BMS at the Integrated Oral Medicine Clinic (CIMO) in Lisbon. Inclusion criteria included a diagnosis of primary BMS based on the International Classification of Orofacial Pain (ICOP) criteria [1], age $\geq$18 years, and complete clinical documentation. Patients with secondary BMS due to local or systemic causes were excluded.

Data collected included sex, age at diagnosis, diagnostic delay (defined as the time from symptom onset to definitive diagnosis), use of psychotropic medications, and self-reported triggering factors. When available, the number of prior appointments and previous diagnoses was also recorded.

Descriptive statistics were used to summarize demographic and clinical characteristics. Associations between variables were assessed using chi-square tests, *t*-tests, and analysis of variance (ANOVA). A significance threshold of $p < 0.05$ was adopted for inferential analyses.

3. Results and Discussion

Among the 300 patients, 82.0% were female. The mean age at diagnosis was 60.3 years for women and 56.6 years for men; this difference was not statistically significant ($p = 0.075$). The overall prevalence of psychotropic drug use was 33.7%, with a significantly higher prevalence among women (42.7%), compared to men (17.8%; $p = 0.002$)—Table 1.

Table 1. Comparison of psychotropic drug use ($p < 0.05$) and mean age at diagnosis ($p > 0.05$) in male and female patients.

	Female	**Male**
Psychotropic drugs (%)	42.7	17.8
Mean of age at diagnosis (years)	60.3	56.6

Stress was the most commonly reported trigger (21.3%)—Figure 1. The mean age at diagnosis—Figure 2—was significantly higher in patients taking psychotropic medications (62.9 years) compared to those not medicated (58.9 years; $p = 0.009$).

Age was inversely associated with diagnostic delay: younger patients were more likely to receive an earlier diagnosis ($p = 0.021$).

Also, of the 300 patients, 42.31% had a diagnostic delay of under a year and a half ($\leq$0.5 Y). However, most of them had a diagnostic delay of up to 5 years (0.5 to 5 Y)—Figure 3.

The findings of this preliminary study align with international literature, highlighting a considerable delay in the diagnosis of BMS and frequent misdiagnoses along the diagnostic pathway [5–7]. This delay remains a significant clinical challenge, as BMS presents with non-specific symptoms that overlap with other oral and systemic conditions [3]. A lack of training and awareness among general physicians and dentists, coupled with the exclusion-based nature of the diagnosis, contributes to diagnostic uncertainty and delays [4]. Additionally, psychotropic medications are commonly prescribed to manage the psychological burden or as part of empirical treatment, although their use often precedes a definitive diagnosis.

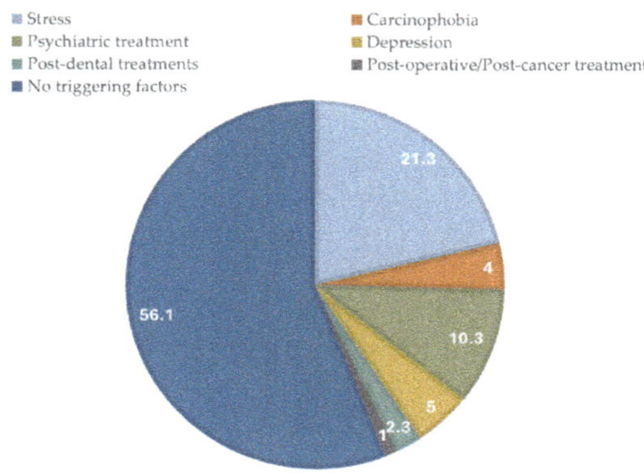

Figure 1. Predominance of different triggering factors in patients with BMS (%).

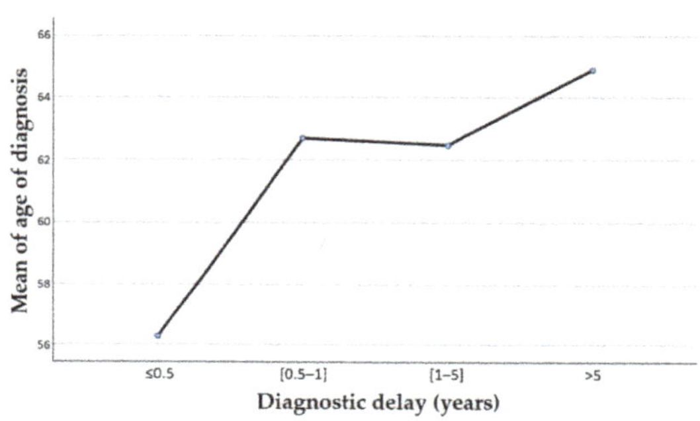

Figure 2. Relationship between age at diagnosis and diagnostic delay ($p < 0.05$).

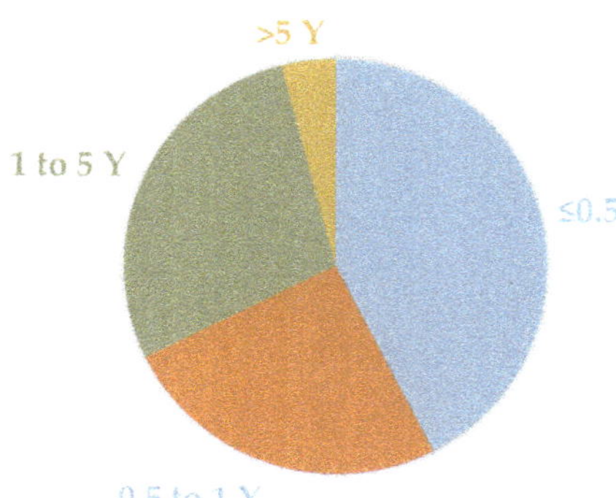

Figure 3. Diagnostic delay in patients with BMS (%).

Our findings further support the association between older age, psychotropic drug use, and prolonged diagnostic delay, in line with other international reports [7]. The data also suggest that younger patients may be more rapidly diagnosed, potentially due to more proactive help-seeking behavior or a higher index of suspicion among clinicians for atypical pain syndromes in younger populations.

Diagnostic delay in BMS not only impacts timely management but is also associated with worsened psychological outcomes and reduced responsiveness to interventions [3]. Patients often express dissatisfaction with their healthcare experiences, reflecting a gap in the delivery of integrated, patient-centered care [5]. Improving diagnostic timelines requires increased education and awareness among healthcare providers, particularly in primary and dental care settings. Early identification protocols and interdisciplinary referral pathways are critical. Patient education and psychological support should also be integrated into routine care for individuals with BMS [6].

4. Conclusions

This study confirms a significant diagnostic delay in Portuguese patients with BMS, particularly among older individuals and those using psychotropic medications. These findings underscore the importance of timely recognition and the need for targeted educational strategies among healthcare professionals. A multidisciplinary approach involving dental, medical, and mental health practitioners is essential to improve outcomes, reduce diagnostic delay, and enhance the quality of life for individuals living with BMS.

Author Contributions: Conceptualization, C.Z. and A.M.A.; methodology, M.V.M.; software, L.P.; validation, C.Z., A.M.A. and P.F.T.; formal analysis, L.P.; investigation, M.V.M.; resources, A.M.A. and P.F.T.; data curation, L.P.; writing—original draft preparation, M.V.M.; writing—review and editing, P.F.T., J.G.E. and A.M.A.; visualization, M.V.M.; supervision, A.M.A.; project administration, C.Z.; funding acquisition, M.V.M. All authors have read and agreed to the published version of the manuscript.

Funding: This research received no external funding.

Institutional Review Board Statement: Ethical review and approval were waived for this study due to its retrospective design. All data were fully anonymized, and patients had been previously informed that their clinical information could be used for research purposes.

Informed Consent Statement: Patient consent was waived due to the retrospective nature of the study. All clinical data were analyzed anonymously, and patients had previously been informed that their data could be used for clinical and research purposes.

Data Availability Statement: The datasets presented in this article are not readily available because the data are part of an ongoing study. Requests to access the datasets should be directed to the corresponding authors.

Conflicts of Interest: The authors declare no conflicts of interest.

References

1. International Headache Society. International Classification of Orofacial Pain, 1st edition (ICOP). *Cephalalgia* **2020**, *40*, 129–221. [CrossRef] [PubMed]
2. Ni Riordain, R.; O'Dwyer, S.; McCreary, C. Burning mouth syndrome—A diagnostic dilemma. *Br. Dent. J.* **2019**, *226*, 835–840. [CrossRef] [PubMed]
3. Mignogna, M.D.; Fedele, S.; Lo Russo, L.; Adamo, D.; Satriano, R.A. Burning mouth syndrome: A review on diagnosis and management. *Oral. Dis.* **2022**, *28*, 5–16. [CrossRef]
4. Galli, F.; Lodi, G.; Sardella, A.; Macchiarelli, G.; Manfredi, M.; Fedele, S.; Carrara, G.; Rossi, R.; Tarsitani, L. Psychological factors in burning mouth syndrome: A systematic review. *J. Oral. Rehabil.* **2023**, *50*, 679–692. [CrossRef]
5. Adamo, D.; Calabria, E.; Canfora, F.; Coppola, N.; Pecoraro, G.; D'Aniello, L.; Aria, M.; Mignogna, M.D.; Leuci, S. Burning mouth syndrome: Analysis of diagnostic delay in 500 patients. *Oral. Dis.* **2024**, *30*, 1–11. [CrossRef] [PubMed]
6. Patil, S.; Patil, P. Burning mouth syndrome: A review. *J Family Med. Prim Care* **2021**, *10*, 2751–2756. [CrossRef]
7. McMillan, R.; Forssell, H.; Buchanan, J.A.; Glenny, A.M.; Zakrzewska, J.M.; Aggarwal, V.R. Interventions for treating burning mouth syndrome. *Cochrane Database Syst Rev.* **2016**, *11*, CD002779. [CrossRef] [PubMed]

medical sciences forum

MDPI

Proceeding Paper

Bespoke Biomarker Combinations for Cancer Survival Prognosis Using Artificial Intelligence on Tumour Transcriptomics †

Ricardo Jorge Pais [1,2,*], Tiago Alexandre Pais [1] and Uraquitan Lima Filho [1]

[1] Bioenhancer Systems Ltd., 407, The Interchange, Manchester SK3 0GF, UK
[2] Egas Moniz Center for Interdisciplinary Research (CiiEM), Egas Moniz School of Health & Science, 2829-511 Almada, Portugal
* Correspondence: rjpais@bioenhancersystems.com

† Presented at the 7th CiiEM International Congress 2025—Empowering One Health to Reduce Social Vulnerabilities, Caparica, Portugal, 2–4 July 2025.

Abstract: Accurate cancer prognosis remains a major challenge, as single gene expression biomarkers often lack clinical reliability, and most ML approaches fail even when considering large gene panels. In this study, we used a novel AutoML framework (O2Pmgen) benchmarked with a well-established framework (TPOT) on TCGA transcriptomic data for breast, lung, and renal cancers to identify small gene panels predictive of patient survival. From 58 EMT-related genes, we found models based on panels of 6–10 genes that outperformed single-marker models and ML models that considered the 58 EMT genes, with performance gains up to 21%. Further, the generated models achieved good predictive power with AUCs of 71–83%. Our results demonstrated that affordable and efficient prognostic tools using small, biologically relevant gene sets can provide better risk stratification in clinical oncology.

Keywords: cancer; prognostic; predictive modelling; machine learning; transcriptomics; artificial intelligence

1. Introduction

Cancer remains one of the leading causes of death globally, with over 10 million deaths recorded annually. While advances in diagnostics and treatment have improved outcomes for many patients, accurately predicting cancer progression and survival remains a significant challenge [1,2]. Current prognostic tools often rely on clinical staging and single-gene biomarkers, frequently lacking the sensitivity, specificity, and predictive power required to guide personalised treatment decisions [3,4]. Prognostic failure can lead to inappropriate therapeutic strategies, delayed interventions, and overall poorer clinical outcomes. In particular, the molecular heterogeneity of tumours is often underrepresented in standard models, limiting their ability to stratify patients effectively by risk [1]. As the field of precision oncology evolves, there is a growing need for robust, cost-effective prognostic tools that can integrate molecular data to enhance clinical decision-making. Recent developments in transcriptomic profiling and artificial intelligence (AI) have opened new avenues for improving cancer prognosis [5–7]. Machine learning and AutoML technologies, when applied to gene expression data, offer a scalable means of identifying complex molecular signatures that are predictive of patient outcomes [8,9]. However, models resulting from such ML frameworks are often considered as "black boxes" and therefore applied to large gene panels to generate highly accurate models [1,10]. This constrains their clinical application, making them expensive and less practical for routine use. In this study, we aim to address these challenges by applying a new AutoML algorithm, O2Pmgen, through the Digital Phenomics platform in an attempt to identify small, biologically meaningful gene panels capable of predicting cancer survival. Using transcriptomic data from The Cancer Genome Atlas (TCGA), we focused on breast, lung, and renal cancers, selecting gene candidates involved in epithelial-to-mesenchymal transition (EMT), a key process in metastasis [11,12].

2. Materials and Methods

Transcriptomic datasets were derived from The Cancer Genome Atlas (TCGA), focusing on primary tumour biopsies from patients with breast (BRCA), lung (LUAD, LUSC), and renal (KICH, KIRC, KIRP) cancers. Transcriptomic data were pre-normalised and obtained as FPKM (fragments per kilobase of transcripts per million mapped reads) expression values from the 2021 Human Protein Atlas transcriptomic profiles [4,13]. On these datasets, a subset of 58 genes was selected based on their roles in epithelial-to-mesenchymal transition (EMT), a hallmark of cancer progression as previously described in [5]. Publicly available data associated with transcriptomics datasets were downloaded from https://www.proteinatlas.org/ (accessed on 10 May 2025). Binarised prognostic outcomes (good/poor) were under the assumption that patients surviving over five years post-diagnosis were labelled as having a good prognosis, while those deceased within two years were classified as poor prognosis, as previously described in [14]. Final datasets consisted of 239 BRCA (40 poor, 199 good), 325 lung (231 poor, 94 good), and 318 renal cancer cases (108 poor, 210 good). All curated datasets were uploaded and made available via the Digital Phenomics platform UIv0.24 (https://digitalphenomics.com, accessed on 10 May 2025).

Three AutoML tools were employed in the same 58-selected genes cancer transcriptomics datasets to develop binary classifiers for prognosis inference: BMfinder, TPOT, and O2Pmgen. BMfinder software (v1.0) was applied for the generation of classifiers based on single-gene abundance thresholds. For each gene, optimal cutoff values were computed to maximise classifier sensitivity across the prognosis classes. The tool applies directionality of the decision rule (above or below the cutoff) depending on whether gene expression was elevated or reduced in poor-prognosis cases. TPOT (Tree-Based Pipeline Optimisation Tool, v0.12.0) was applied using a genetic programming framework to evolve optimal ML pipelines [8] For each dataset, TPOT performed 100 evolutionary generations with a population of 50 models, using 5-fold cross-validation and ROC-AUC as the optimisation criterion. Model generation using TPOT and BMfinder was executed on a 16-core VPS environment running custom Python 3.8 scripts. O2Pmgen (v1.1) was executed via the Digital Phenomics platform [14]. This proprietary AI-driven AutoML tool uses an evolution-inspired multi-objective optimisation algorithm to identify optimal combinations of gene expression patterns [14]. The algorithm was constrained to train on <50% of the dataset, retaining the remainder for testing. Models incorporated both directionality (up/down regulation) and binary presence logic of multiple biomarkers on a scoring function, as previously described in [14].

Classifier performance was assessed using Receiver Operating Characteristic Area Under the Curve (ROC-AUC), sensitivity, and specificity metrics computed using the software tool ROCplot version 1.0 [14]. Optimal sensitivity (True Positive Rate) and specificity (True Negative Rate) were computed using ROCplot on the entire dataset to ensure an accurate and deterministic calculation of model performance metrics without requiring confidence intervals.

3. Results

Using autoML approaches, we obtained a bespoke predictive model for the prognosis of each cancer type. NFKB2, PTK2 and TGFB1 genes were identified as single bespoke predictive biomarkers for breast, lung and renal cancers, respectively. Bespoke combinations of 10 biomarkers that maximise the predictive capacity were identified for breast cancer and combinations of 6 biomarkers for the remaining cancer types (Figure 1). Breast, lung, and renal cancer types exhibited distinct gene expression patterns and shared only two genes (ILK and EGF) between different cancer types. Interestingly, none of the identified single bespoke biomarkers were present in the bespoke combinations.

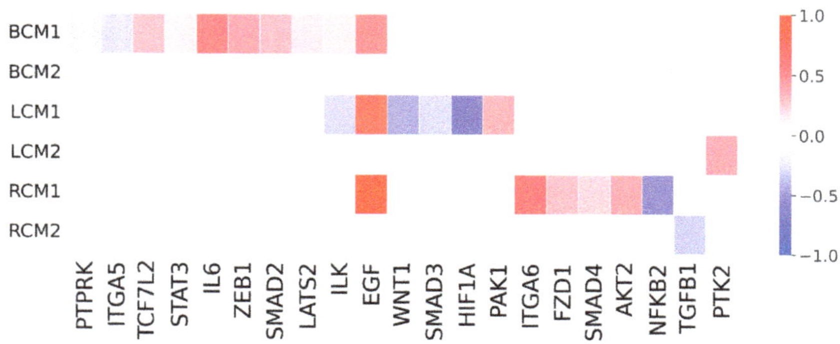

Figure 1. Predicted single biomarkers and combinations of biomarkers identified for breast, lung and renal cancers. Gene names are indicated on the *x*-axis, and the normalised degree of variation between cancer survival medians and controls is represented on the *y*-axis. BCM1, LCM1 and RCM1 indicate the predictive combination of biomarkers for breast, lung and renal cancers, respectively. BCM2, LCM2 and RCM2 indicate the single predictive biomarkers for breast, lung and renal cancers, respectively. Gene downregulations in expression are depicted by negative numbers represented by a blue gradient scale, and up-regulations by positive numbers in a red gradient scale. Null values in white represent that the gene was not identified as a predictive biomarker.

Performance evaluation of the generated predictive models (Table 1) showed substantial improvement of performance metrics (AUC, sensitivity and specificity) of models composed of combinations of biomarkers (O2Pmgen-derived) in comparison with the single biomarker approach (BMfinder-derived). Models derived by autoML using all genes (TPOT-derived) showed equivalent improvements on sensitivity but only mild improvements on the AUC and specificity.

Table 1. Performance of the models generated using different ML approaches.

Cancer Type	Model	Software tool	AUC	Sensitivity	Specificity
Breast	BCM1	O2Pmgen v1.1	83%	95%	63%
	BCM2	BMfinder v1.0	62%	84%	42%
	BCM3	TPOT v0.12.0	65%	95%	40%
Lung	LCM1	O2Pmgen v1.1	75%	81%	61%
	LCM2	BMfinder v1.0	60%	71%	40%
	LCM3	TPOT v0.12.0	63%	79%	50%
Renal	RCM1	O2Pmgen v1.1	71%	81%	60%
	RCM2	BMfinder v1.0	62%	73%	41%
	RCM3	TPOT v0.12.0	68%	82%	63%

4. Discussion

The results of this study underscore the potential of AI-driven approaches for identifying bespoke predictive models and clinically relevant biomarkers. Notably, we demonstrated that employing advanced modelling strategies such as O2Pmgen, which iteratively searches, evaluates, and selects optimal biomarker combinations, can lead to substantial gains in predictive performance. Across the three cancer types analysed, this approach yielded up to a 21% increase in AUC compared with both a widely used AutoML framework (TPOT) and the best-performing single-biomarker classifier.

The obtained sensitivities and specificities suggest that O2Pmgen tends to generate models with higher specificity than traditional approaches, explaining the observed gains in predictive power. These models consistently showed improved specificity relative to baseline models, often without a corresponding loss in sensitivity. The algorithm tends to prioritise specificity, potentially reducing false positive rates. In clinical contexts, this may be advantageous where the goal is to minimise overtreatment or unnecessary follow-up of patients incorrectly identified as high risk. However, such specificity could lead to under-identification of true positive cases, which may be unacceptable in settings where early detection is critical. The clinical appropriateness of this trade-off depends on the intended application and patient population.

Importantly, the predictive models generated by O2Pmgen were based on compact and biologically interpretable gene panels, offering a valuable opportunity for developing cost-effective and practical prognostic tools to support clinical decision-making in oncology. Furthermore, the selected gene combinations exhibited distinct patterns of upregulation and downregulation of signalling components specific to each cancer type, suggesting the presence of tumour-specific molecular signatures associated with favourable prognosis.

Interestingly, the expression patterns identified align with transcriptomic and signalling features characteristic of mesenchymal-like cancer cells, while being incompatible with highly invasive or metastable hybrid phenotypes [11,15]. These findings support the hypothesis that the gene panels discovered through our AI-guided approach reflect stable, less aggressive tumour states and correlate with improved clinical outcomes.

Although the models showed promising performance, limitations should be acknowledged. These include reliance on retrospective TCGA data without independent validation, potential bias from unbalanced datasets (notably in breast cancer), and restriction to 58 genes, which may limit broader model optimisation. Thus, results should be interpreted cautiously and viewed primarily as a qualitative comparison across AutoML approaches.

5. Conclusions

This work demonstrates that autoML strategies for developing models based on finding optimal combinations of small gene sets can outperform the predictive power of larger, less practical panels. The findings highlight the potential for affordable, scalable, and clinically applicable prognostic tools that support personalised oncology and improved patient management. As next steps, we aim to extend this approach by exploring the full transcriptomic space to identify improved gene set combinations. Additionally, external validation using independent datasets will be pursued to strengthen the clinical relevance and generalisability of the models.

Author Contributions: Conceptualisation, R.J.P. and U.L.F.; methodology, R.J.P. and U.L.F.; software, R.J.P. and U.L.F.; validation, T.A.P.; formal analysis, T.A.P.; data curation, T.A.P.; writing—original draft preparation, R.J.P.; writing—review and editing, R.J.P.; supervision, R.J.P. All authors have read and agreed to the published version of the manuscript.

Funding: This research was supported by the UK Government through the Innovation Navigator—Flexible Fund grant GMBS-FF-180057, which was awarded for the development of the Digital Phenomics platform.

Institutional Review Board Statement: Not applicable.

Informed Consent Statement: Not applicable.

Data Availability Statement: All data in this research is available at https://digitalphenomics.com, accessed on 10 May 2025.

Acknowledgments: The authors acknowledge Bioenhancer Systems Ltd. for supporting the resources necessary to conduct the analysis and maintain the tools online. The authors also acknowledge the Manchester Growth Business Innovation Hub for helping with grant acquisition and management, which gave rise to this work.

Conflicts of Interest: R. Pais declares a potential conflict of interest as he is the director of Bioenhancer Systems. U. Filho and T. Pais declare no conflict of interest.

References

1. Kourou, K.; Exarchos, K.P.; Papaloukas, C.; Sakaloglou, P.; Exarchos, T.; Fotiadis, D.I. Applied Machine Learning in Cancer Research: A Systematic Review for Patient Diagnosis, Classification and Prognosis. *Comput. Struct. Biotechnol. J.* **2021**, *19*, 5546–5555. [CrossRef]
2. Boeri, C.; Chiappa, C.; Galli, F.; De Berardinis, V.; Bardelli, L.; Carcano, G.; Rovera, F. Machine Learning Techniques in Breast Cancer Prognosis Prediction: A Primary Evaluation. *Cancer Med.* **2020**, *9*, 3234–3243. [CrossRef]
3. Šutić, M.; Vukić, A.; Baranašić, J.; Försti, A.; Džubur, F.; Samaržija, M.; Jakopović, M.; Brčić, L.; Knežević, J. Diagnostic, Predictive, and Prognostic Biomarkers in Non-Small Cell Lung Cancer (NSCLC) Management. *J. Pers. Med.* **2021**, *11*, 1102. [CrossRef] [PubMed]
4. Pontén, F.; Jirström, K.; Uhlen, M. The Human Protein Atlas—A Tool for Pathology. *J. Pathol.* **2008**, *216*, 387–393. [CrossRef] [PubMed]
5. Pais, R.J.; Lopes, F.; Parreira, I.; Silva, M.; Silva, M.; Moutinho, M.G. Predicting Cancer Prognostics from Tumour Transcriptomics Using an Auto Machine Learning Approach. *Med. Sci. Forum* **2023**, *22*, 6.
6. Yang, D.; Ma, X.; Song, P. A Prognostic Model of Non Small Cell Lung Cancer Based on TCGA and ImmPort Databases. *Sci. Rep.* **2022**, *12*, 437. [CrossRef] [PubMed]
7. Wu, G.; Xu, Y.; Han, C.; Wang, Z.; Li, J.; Wang, Q.; Che, X. Identification of a Prognostic Risk Signature of Kidney Renal Clear Cell Carcinoma Based on Regulating the Immune Response Pathway Exploration. *J. Oncol.* **2020**, *2020*, 6657013. [CrossRef] [PubMed]
8. Le, T.T.; Fu, W.; Moore, J.H. Scaling Tree-Based Automated Machine Learning to Biomedical Big Data with a Feature Set Selector. *Bioinformatics* **2020**, *36*, 250–256. [CrossRef] [PubMed]
9. Telikani, A.; Gandomi, A.H.; Tahmassebi, A.; Banzhaf, W. Evolutionary Machine Learning: A Survey. *ACM Comput. Surv.* **2021**, *54*, 161. [CrossRef]
10. Roman-Naranjo, P.; Parra-Perez, A.M.; Lopez-Escamez, J.A. A Systematic Review on Machine Learning Approaches in the Diagnosis and Prognosis of Rare Genetic Diseases. *J. Biomed. Inform.* **2023**, *143*, 104429. [CrossRef] [PubMed]
11. Liao, T.-T.; Yang, M.-H. Hybrid Epithelial/Mesenchymal State in Cancer Metastasis: Clinical Significance and Regulatory Mechanisms. *Cells* **2020**, *9*, 623. [CrossRef] [PubMed]
12. Garg, M. Epithelial, Mesenchymal and Hybrid Epithelial/Mesenchymal Phenotypes and Their Clinical Relevance in Cancer Metastasis. *Expert Rev. Mol. Med.* **2017**, *19*, e3. [CrossRef]
13. Uhlen, M.; Zhang, C.; Lee, S.; Sjöstedt, E.; Fagerberg, L.; Bidkhori, G.; Benfeitas, R.; Arif, M.; Liu, Z.; Edfors, F.; et al. A Pathology Atlas of the Human Cancer Transcriptome. *Science* **2017**, 357. [CrossRef] [PubMed]
14. Filho, U.L.; Pais, T.A.; Pais, R.J. Facilitating "Omics" for Phenotype Classification Using a User-Friendly AI-Driven Platform: Application in Cancer Prognostics. *BioMedInformatics* **2023**, *3*, 1071–1082. [CrossRef]
15. Pais, R.J. Simulation of Multiple Microenvironments Shows a Pivot Role of RPTPs on the Control of Epithelial-to-Mesenchymal Transition. *Biosystems* **2020**, *198*, 104268. [CrossRef] [PubMed]

medical sciences forum

MDPI

Proceeding Paper

Parental Satisfaction in Short-Stay Pediatric Emergency Unit: A Cross-Sectional, Descriptive and Observational Study †

Vanessa Antunes [1,*], Paula Pereira [2], Tatiana Cardoso [2], Célia Pereira [2], Miguel Ladeira [2], Ricardo Antunes [1] and Fernanda Loureiro [3]

1 Centro de Investigação Interdisciplinar Egas Moniz (CiiEM), Escola Superior de Saúde Egas Moniz, 2829-551 Caparica, Portugal
2 Unidade de Urgência Pediátrica, Hospital Garcia de Orta, 2805-251 Almada, Portugal
3 Centro de Investigação Interdisciplinar em Saúde (CIIS), Universidade Católica Portuguesa, 1649-023 Lisboa, Portugal; floureiro@ucp.pt
* Correspondence: vantunes@egasmoniz.edu.pt

† Presented at the 7th CiiEM International Congress 2025—Empowering One Health to Reduce Social Vulnerabilities, Caparica, Portugal, 2–4 July 2025.

Abstract: This study evaluated parental satisfaction with nursing care in a pediatric emergency department short-stay unit. Using the Citizen Satisfaction with Nursing Care Scale, 205 parents of hospitalized children participated in a descriptive, cross-sectional study. Results showed consistently high satisfaction, regardless of parental sociodemographic characteristics. While parents of newborns and employed parents showed slightly higher satisfaction, differences were not statistically significant. These trends suggest areas for further qualitative research to better understand parental expectations. The findings highlight the importance of ongoing evaluation and structured feedback to maintain high-quality, responsive nursing care in pediatric emergency settings.

Keywords: parental satisfaction; hospitals; pediatric; nursing care; child; hospitalized

1. Introduction

Customer satisfaction is a key indicator of healthcare quality, reflecting the extent to which services meet patient and family expectations [1]. Within hospital settings, satisfaction with nursing care plays a pivotal role in shaping overall satisfaction with the hospital experience, representing the most influential dimension [2]. High levels of satisfaction are closely associated with improved adherence to treatment and care plans, as well as increased likelihood of patients and families recommending or returning to the healthcare facility—making satisfaction a valuable metric for assessing care quality [3]. In the context of nursing care, satisfaction is defined as "a personal opinion that compares perceived needs, expectations of care and experiences of care received in the professional, personal and environmental domains" [4] (p. 28). To capture this multifaceted concept, a variety of validated measurement instruments have been developed and are well-documented in the literature [5]. During a child's hospital stay, parents—especially mothers—are typically the primary companions and serve as key respondents in satisfaction assessments [6,7]. While parental satisfaction is relevant across all pediatric care settings, including emergency, inpatient, and intensive care units, studies in the national context—particularly within pediatric emergency services remain scarce.

Given this gap, the present study aims to evaluate parental satisfaction with nursing care provided to children admitted to short-stay units in the pediatric emergency department (PED). By identifying how parents perceive nursing care in this specific setting,

 https://doi.org/10.3390/msf2025037021

the study seeks to contribute to the evidence base and support future improvements in clinical practice.

2. Materials and Methods

2.1. Study Design

This is a cross-sectional, descriptive and observational study with a quantitative approach. We adhere to the reporting guidelines of the Enhancing Quality and Transparency of Health Research (EQUATOR) network. More specifically, we followed the Strengthening the Reporting of Observational Studies in Epidemiology (STROBE) checklist. The study was registered on 30 March 2022 at Open Science Framework (https://osf.io/mabgv/ accessed on 7 May 2025).

2.2. Setting and Participants

The study was applied in a PED at a regional public hospital in Portugal. The PED includes two areas: an external area for initial assessment and care, and an internal short-stay inpatient unit (SSIU), where children remain under observation for up to 48 h. In this setting, each child is continuously accompanied by a caregiver, typically the mother. Data were collected over six months (June to December 2023) from parents or caregivers at the time of discharge. Inclusion criteria were being the primary companion during the child's stay in the SSIU, sufficient proficiency in written and spoken Portuguese, and informed consent to participate.

2.3. Variables and Measurement

Independent variables included socio-demographic variables regarding the children (sex, age, triage wristband color, length of stay) and the carer (sex, age, educational level, employment status-employed/unemployed—and occupational class according to the National Classification of Occupations). Dependent variables included satisfaction with nursing care measured through an instrument entitled Citizen Satisfaction with Nursing Care Scale. This scale was originally designed to be applied in primary care setting; however, it has already been adapted and validated to be applied to parents of hospitalized children [8]. It includes two subscales: Nursing Care Experiences ([NCE] 28 items rated on a seven-item Likert scale) and Opinions on Nursing Care ([ONC] 19 items rated on a five-item Likert scale). To test reliability, we assessed internal consistency through Cronbach's alpha coefficients and obtained values of 0.979 and 0.980, respectively.

2.4. Study Size and Bias

A convenience sampling method was used. While this approach facilitated access to participants, it may introduce selection bias and limit generalizability. To minimize researcher bias, the team was divided: one subgroup administered the data collection, while another conducted the statistical analysis. This separation aimed to enhance objectivity and reduce the influence of researcher expectations on data interpretation.

2.5. Quantitative Variables and Statistical Methods

The data were organized and analyzed using IBM SPSS Statistics® for Windows (v. 29.0; IBM Corp., New York, NY, USA). Descriptive statistics were used to summarize categorical variables as frequencies and percentages and continuous variables as mean and standard deviation. For inferential analysis, the assumption of normal distribution was assessed using the Kolmogorov–Smirnov test, and the homogeneity of variances was verified using Levene's test. Subsequently, statistical analyses were conducted using Student's *t*-test and one-way analysis of variance (ANOVA). A *p*-value ≤ 0.05 was considered statistically significant.

3. Results and Discussion

A total of 205 parents participated in this study. Most of the children were male, younger in age, and admitted in urgent situations—findings consistent with the existing literature [9]. Most parents were female, aged $\geq$ 30, and employed. Overall, they reported high satisfaction with nursing care. Interestingly, no statistically significant associations were found between satisfaction levels and parental sociodemographic characteristics as shown in Table 1. This suggests that satisfaction with nursing care in the PED setting may be more closely linked to the nature of the interaction and the quality of care rather than individual or cultural variables. Previous literature supports this conclusion, emphasizing that parental satisfaction is strongly associated with interpersonal communication, timely interventions, and perceived competence of nursing staff rather than socio-demographic factors [10].

Table 1. Participant socio-demographic characteristics and average results from scale application.

Socio-Demographic Characteristics		n	%	NCS (1–7)			ONC (1–5)		
				M	SD	*p*	M	SD	*p*
Children sex	Male	105	52.5	6.5	0.54	0.871	4.5	0.58	0.851
	Female	95	57.5	6.5	0.60		4.6	0.63	
Children age	Newborn	8	4	6.7	0.44	0.657	4.8	0.35	0.450
	Infant	62	31	6.4	0.57		4.4	0.66	
	Toddler	28	14	6.5	0.48		4.5	0.50	
	Preschool	19	9.5	6.4	0.77		4.5	0.62	
	School age	35	17.5	6.6	0.54		4.7	0.65	
	Adolescent	48	24	6.5	0.57		4.6	0.59	
Wristband color assigned in the PED	Blue	1	0.6	6.4		0.98	4.0		0.936
	Green	28	16.1	6.4	0.61		4.5	0.64	
	Yellow	46	26.4	6.4	0.61		4.5	0.56	
	Orange	90	51.7	6.5	0.54		4.5	0.66	
	Red	9	5.2	6.4	0.57		4.6	0.58	
Length of hospital stay (hours)	≤12 h	49	25.9	6.5	0.55	0.731	4.5	0.64	0.746
	13–24 h	102	54	6.5	0.55		4.5	0.61	
	≥25 h	38	20.1	6.4	0.65		4.6	0.55	
Sex of carer	Male	32	16.2	6.5	0.48	0.821	4.5	0.59	0.898
	Female	166	83.8	6.5	0.55		4.6	0.60	
Carer age (years)	≤29 years	40	20.1	6.5	0.56	0.908	4.4	0.69	0.207
	30–39 years	92	46.2	6.5	0.52		4.6	0.53	
	40–49 years	53	26.6	6.4	0.64		4.5	0.68	
	≥50 years	14	7	6.5	0.59		4.7	0.47	

Table 1. *Cont.*

Socio-Demographic Characteristics		n	%	NCS (1–7)			ONC (1–5)		
				M	SD	*p*	M	SD	*p*
Carer's education (years)	Up to 6 years	12	6.9	6.3	0.58	0.161	4.7	0.44	0.029
	7–9 years	36	20.6	6.3	0.72		4.3	0.73	
	10–12 years	84	48	6.5	0.52		4.6	0.51	
	Higher education	43	24.6	6.5	0.45		4.6	0.58	
Employment status	Employed	160	83.3	6.5	0.49	0.096	4.6	0.54	0.301
	Unemployed	32	16.7	6.3	0.70		4.5	0.67	
Socio-Professional Classes	Professions in the Armed Forces	3	1.9	6.5	0.37	0.171	4.7	0.26	0.688
	Representatives of executive bodies, directors and managers	3	1.9	6.9	0.09		5.0	0.06	
	Specialists in intellectual and scientific activities	49	30.8	6.6	0.43		4.6	0.58	
	Technicians and mid-level professions	24	15.1	6.6	0.47		4.5	0.57	
	Administrative staff	15	9.4	6.6	0.36		4.7	0.33	
	Personal service, security and sales workers	36	22.6	6.6	0.43		4.7	0.55	
	Skilled agricultural, fishing and forestry workers	1	0.6	6.7			4.9	0.6	
	Skilled construction workers and craftsmen	3	1.9	6.4	0.52		4.3	1.9	
	Plant and machine operators and assembly workers	4	2.5	6.7	0.39		4.5	2.5	
	Unqualified workers	21	13.2	6.2	0.79		4.4	13.2	

Although no statistically significant associations were found between satisfaction scores and parental sociodemographic characteristics, an observable pattern emerged—particularly among parents of newborns, who reported the highest satisfaction levels on both the NCS and ONC scales. While these findings must be interpreted with caution due to the lack of statistical significance, the consistency of the pattern suggests a potential relationship that warrants further investigation. Such exploratory findings, although not conclusive, may help to generate hypotheses for future studies with greater statistical power or complementary methodologies. The heightened sensitivity and emotional needs of parents during early age might influence their perception of care. This finding aligns with a study by Kwiatosz-Muc et al. [11], who reported that the age of the hospitalized child did not significantly affect parental satisfaction, but that parents of younger children, particularly infants, often express heightened emotional responses and gratitude for attentive nursing care. Although the difference was not statistically significant, employed parents reported higher satisfaction levels compared to unemployed parents. This finding suggests that employment status may influence perceptions of nursing care quality. Employed parents might value efficiency, clear communication, and structured care processes more due to their limited availability and work responsibilities. This aligns with previous studies indicating that socioeconomic and professional status can shape expectations and satisfaction with healthcare services [12]. Qualitative approaches could provide deeper insight into how employment status affects parental satisfaction. From a clinical perspective, the consistently high satisfaction scores are encouraging and reflect positively on the PED nursing staff. Nonetheless, the lack of statistically significant differentiation across groups might also suggest a ceiling effect of the measurement instrument or a homogenous sample in terms of healthcare satisfaction. Future research could benefit from using mixed methods approaches to capture more nuanced parental experiences and identify subtle areas for improvement.

4. Conclusions

The findings revealed high levels of parental satisfaction with nursing care in the PED short-stay unit, regardless of sociodemographic background, indicating a generally positive perception of care quality. Although no statistically significant differences were observed, certain non-significant patterns—such as higher satisfaction among employed parents and those of newborns—may point to areas of interest for future research. These exploratory observations should be interpreted with caution, but they may help guide the design of studies with larger samples or different methodological approaches. Incorporating structured feedback mechanisms into routine care could further support ongoing improvements in the quality of pediatric emergency nursing.

Author Contributions: Conceptualization, F.L., P.P., T.C., C.P., M.L., R.A. and V.A.; methodology, F.L., P.P., T.C., C.P., M.L., R.A. and V.A.; formal analysis, F.L., R.A. and V.A.; investigation, P.P., T.C., C.P. and M.L.; resources, F.L., P.P., T.C., C.P., M.L., R.A. and V.A.; data curation, F.L., P.P., T.C., C.P., M.L., R.A. and V.A.; writing—original draft preparation, V.A.; writing—review and editing, F.L., P.P., T.C., C.P., M.L., R.A. and V.A.; supervision, F.L.; project administration, F.L. All authors have read and agreed to the published version of the manuscript.

Funding: This research received no external funding.

Institutional Review Board Statement: The study was conducted in accordance with the Declaration of Helsinki and approved by the Ethics Committee for Health of Hospital Garcia de Orta (protocol code 28/2023, approved on 17 April 2023).

Informed Consent Statement: Informed consent was obtained from all subjects.

Data Availability Statement: Data is available on reasonable request to the corresponding author.

Acknowledgments: The authors express their gratitude to the parents who took part in the study.

Conflicts of Interest: The authors declare no conflicts of interest.

References

1. Ali, J.; Jusoh, A.; Idris, N.; Nor, K.M. Healthcare service quality and patient satisfaction: A conceptual framework. *Int. J. Qual. Reliab. Manag.* **2024**, *41*, 608–627. [CrossRef]
2. Karaca, A.; Durna, Z. Patient satisfaction with the quality of nursing care. *Nurs. Open* **2019**, *6*, 535–545. Available online: http://www.ncbi.nlm.nih.gov/pubmed/30918704 (accessed on 7 May 2025). [CrossRef] [PubMed]
3. Ferreira, D.C.; Vieira, I.; Pedro, M.I.; Caldas, P.; Varela, M. Patient Satisfaction with Healthcare Services and the Techniques Used for its Assessment: A Systematic Literature Review and a Bibliometric Analysis. *Healthcare* **2023**, *11*, 639. Available online: https://pmc.ncbi.nlm.nih.gov/articles/PMC10001171/ (accessed on 7 May 2025). [CrossRef] [PubMed]
4. Loureiro, F.; Charepe, Z. Patient Satisfaction with Nursing Care in Hospital: Concept Analysis. *Cad. De Saúde* **2018**, *10*, 23–29. [CrossRef]
5. Loureiro, F.M.; Antunes, V. Instruments to evaluate hospitalised children parents' satisfaction with nursing care: A scoping review. *BMJ Paediatr. Open* **2022**, *6*, e001568. [CrossRef] [PubMed]
6. Loureiro, F.; Figueiredo, M.H.; Charepe, Z. Nursing care satisfaction from school-aged children's perspective: An integrative review. *Int. J. Nurs. Pract.* **2019**, *25*, e12764. [CrossRef] [PubMed]
7. Mucuk, S.P.; Cimke, S.R.N.; Mucuk, S.P.; Cimke, S.R.N. Mothers' Participation in the Hospitalized Children's Care and their Satis-faction. *Int. J. Caring Sci.* **2017**, *10*, 1643–1651. Available online: http://www.internationaljournalofcaringsciences.org/docs/59_1-cimke_original_10_3.pdf (accessed on 7 May 2025).
8. Loureiro, F.; Araújo, B.; Charepe, Z. Validation of the Citizen Satisfaction with Nursing Care Scale for parents of hospitalized children. *Rev. De Enferm. Ref.* **2021**, *5*, 1–8. [CrossRef]

9. Neuman, M.I.; Alpern, E.R.; Hall, M.; Kharbanda, A.B.; Shah, S.S.; Freedman, S.B.; Aronson, P.L.; Florin, T.A.; Mistry, R.D.; Berry, J.G. Characteristics of Recurrent Utilization in Pediatric Emergency Departments. *Pediatrics* **2014**, *134*, e1025–e1031. Available online: https://pubmed.ncbi.nlm.nih.gov/25225134/ (accessed on 26 May 2025). [PubMed]
10. Sam, C.J.; Arunachalam, P.A.; Manivasagan, S.; Surya, T. Parental Satisfaction with Pediatric Day-Care Surgery and its Determinants in a Tertiary Care Hospital. *J. Indian Assoc. Pediatr. Surg.* **2017**, *22*, 226. Available online: https://pmc.ncbi.nlm.nih.gov/articles/PMC5615897/ (accessed on 29 May 2025). [CrossRef] [PubMed]
11. Kruszecka-Krówka, A.; Smoleń, E.; Cepuch, G.; Piskorz-Ogórek, K.; Perek, M.; Gniadek, A. Determinants of Parental Satisfaction with Nursing Care in Paediatric Wards—A Preliminary Report. *Int. J. Environ. Res. Public Health* **2019**, *16*, 1774. Available online: https://www.mdpi.com/1660-4601/16/10/1774/htm (accessed on 26 May 2025). [CrossRef] [PubMed]
12. Aloh, H.E.; Onwujekwe, O.E.; Aloh, O.G.; Okoronkwo, I.L.; Nweke, C.J. Impact of socioeconomic status on patient experience on quality of care for ambulatory healthcare services in tertiary hospitals in Southeast Nigeria. *BMC Health Serv. Res.* **2020**, *20*, 473. Available online: https://pubmed.ncbi.nlm.nih.gov/32456633/ (accessed on 29 May 2025). [CrossRef] [PubMed]

MDPI AG
Grosspeteranlage 5
4052 Basel
Switzerland
Tel.: +41 61 683 77 34

Medical Sciences Forum Editorial Office
E-mail: msf@mdpi.com
www.mdpi.com/journal/msf

www.ingramcontent.com/pod-product-compliance
Lightning Source LLC
Chambersburg PA
CBHW040717270926
51850CB00023B/2776
9783725856312